@Copyright 2020 By Patrick Pearse **All Rights reserved**

This report aims to provide precise and sound data on the point and problem secured. It was possible for the distributor not to make bookkeeping, to be requested in the call.

The Declaration of Principles accepted and supported by the American Bar Association Committee and the Publishers and Associations Committee.

Not the least bit is permissible for any piece of this report to be replicated,copied or transmitted in either electronic methods or the group.The recording of this distribution is carefully refused, and any capacity in this report is not allowed unless the distributor has composed the authorization. All rights.

The data in this is conveyed,to be truthful and predictable,inasmuch as any danger, to absent mind or something else,is a single and articulate duty of a beneficiary peruser through use or maltreatment of any methods, procedures, or bearings embedded within it.No lawful obligation or default shall be made against the distributor for any reparation,damage,or money misfortune due to the information in this,either directly or implicitly.

Any copyrights not held by the seller are asserted by individual authors.

The data in this document is only available for educational purposes and is all-inclusive.The data are entered without a contract or confirmation of assurance.

The marks used shall be without consent, and the mark shall be distributed without the consent or support of the proprietor.All trademarks and trademarks in this book are for explanation only and are clearly held by owners who are not associated with the record.

Table of Contents

Chapter 1: All You Need to Know About Diabetes 5

    What is Diabetes? 5

    What is Type 1 Diabetes? 5

    What are the Warning Signs of Type 1 Diabetes? 6

    Type 1 Diabetes Treatment 6

    What is Type 2 Diabetes? 7

    What are the Warning Signs of Type 2 Diabetes? 7

    Type 2 Diabetes Treatment 8

Chapter 2 Things You Need to Know About Meal Prepping 8

    The Difference Between Meal Planning and Meal Prep 8

    The 7 Benefits of Meal Prepping 8

        Temptation Removal 8

        Total Control 9

        Hunger Manager 9

        Timesaver 9

        Money Saver 9

        Waste Eliminator 9

        Stress Remover 10

    10 Tips for Easy Meal Prep 10

        Start small. 10

        Keep it simple, stupid. 10

        Make a list, check it twice. 11

        Make cleanup a breeze. 11

        Practice those knife skills. 11

        Order matters. 11

        Frozen is fine. 12

        Prevent waste. 12

        Freezing and reheating. 12

        Food safety. 12

Breakfast Recipes 13

    Bell Pepper Pancakes 13

    Sweet Potato Waffles 13

    Quinoa Bread 14

    Tofu Scramble 14

    Apple Omelet 15

    Veggie Frittata 16

    Chicken & Sweet Potato Hash 17

    MINI VEGGIE QUICHE 18

    SHAKSHUKA 19

    HEALTHY GRANOLA 20

    CINNAMON OATMEAL MUFFINS WITH APPLE 21

    VEGGIE OMELET 22

    Spinach Scramble 23

    Breakfast Parfait 23

    Asparagus & Cheese Omelet 24

Lunch Recipes 25

    TORTILLA CHICKEN SOUP 25

CHICKEN BROCCOLI SALAD 26

BLACK BEAN SALAD 27

KALE SALAD WITH LEMON DRESSING 28

CARROT GINGER SOUP 29

SHRIMP SALAD 30

CRISPY TOFU 31

SPINACH SOUP WITH PESTO & CHICKEN 32

Asian Cold Noodle Salad 33

Chicken Tortilla Soup 34

Dinner Recipes 35

  FRENCH LENTILS 35

  CHICKEN FAJITAS 36

  VEGGIE RICE 37

  GRILLED TUNA KEBABS 38

  SPICY TURKEY TACOS 39

  LIME QUINOA WITH CILANTRO 40

  POTATOES WITH ROASTED VEGGIES 41

  MUSHROOM STROGANOFF 42

  Almond-Crusted Salmon 43

  Chicken & Veggie Bowl with Brown Rice 44

Meat Recipes 45

  Beef Salad 45

  Beef Curry 46

  Beef with Barley & Veggies 47

  Beef with Broccoli 48

  Pan Grilled Steak 49

  Lamb Stew 50

  Lamb Curry 51

  Meatballs in Tomato Gravy 52

  Spiced Leg of Lamb 53

  Baked Lamb & Spinach 54

  Pork Salad 55

  Pork with Bell Peppers 55

  Roasted Pork Shoulder 56

  Pork Chops in Peach Glaze 57

  Ground Pork with Spinach 58

Poultry Recipes 59

  Chicken with Chickpeas 59

  Chicken & Broccoli Bake 60

  Meatballs Curry 61

  Chicken, Oats & Chickpeas Meatloaf 62

  Herbed Turkey Breast 63

  Turkey with Lentils 64

Vegetarian Recipes 65

  Baked Beans 65

  Spicy Black Beans 66

  Lentils Chili 67

  Quinoa in Tomato Sauce 68

  Grains Combo 68

  Barley Pilaf 69

  Baked Veggies Combo 70

  Mixed Veggie Salad 71

  Tofu with Brussels Sprout 72

  Beans, Walnuts & Veggie Burgers 73

Side Recipes 74

  Spicy Spinach 74

Herbed Asparagus 74
Lemony Brussels Sprout 75
Gingered Cauliflower 75
Roasted Broccoli 76
Garlicky Cabbage 76
Stir Fried Zucchini 77
Green Beans with Tomatoes 77
French Green Beans 78
Roasted Summer Squash 78
Veggie Mash 79
Mushroom Medley 79

Fish And Seafood Recipes 80
Salmon Soup 80
Salmon & Shrimp Stew 81
Salmon Curry 82
Salmon with Bell Peppers 83
Shrimp Salad 84
Shrimp & Veggies Curry 85
Shrimp with Zucchini 86
Shrimp with Broccoli 86
Grilled Salmon with Ginger Sauce 87

Dessert Recipes 88
SUGAR FREE BUCKEYE BALLS 88
PEANUT BUTTER COOKIES 89
CHOCOLATE FUDGE 90
LOW-CARB CHEESECAKE 90
Chocolate & Raspberry Ice Cream 91
Mocha Pops 91
Choco Banana Bites 92
Blueberries with Yogurt 92
Fruit Kebab 93
Roasted Mangoes 93
Figs with Yogurt 94
Grilled Peaches 94
Fruit Salad 95

30 - day meal plan 96

Chapter 1: All You Need to Know About Diabetes

What is Diabetes?

Diabetes is a serious condition that causes higher than normal blood sugar levels. Diabetes occurs when your body cannot make or effectively use its own insulin, a hormone made by special cells in the pancreas called islets (eye-lets). Insulin serves as a "key" to open your cells, to allow the sugar (glucose) from the food you eat to enter. Then, your body uses that glucose for energy.

But with diabetes, several major things can go wrong to cause diabetes. Type 1 and type 2 diabetes are the most common forms of the disease, but there are also other kinds, such as gestational diabetes, which occurs during pregnancy, as well as other forms.

What is Type 1 Diabetes?

Type 1 diabetes, previously known as juvenile diabetes, is the most severe form of the disease. About 5% of people who have diabetes have type 1 diabetes, or insulin-dependent diabetes. Type 1 diabetes has also been called juvenile diabetes becuse it usually develops in children and teenagers. But people of all ages can develop type 1 diabetes.

In type 1 diabetes, the body's immune system attacks the insulin-producing islet cells in the pancreas. The islet cells sense glucose in the blood and produce the right amount of insulin to normalize blood sugars. This attack on the body's own cells is known as autoimmune disease. Scientists are not sure why the autoimmune attack happens.

But once the insulin-producing cells are destroyed, a person can no longer produce their own insulin. Without insulin, there is no "key." So, the sugar stays in the blood and builds up. As a result, the body's cells starve. And, if left untreated, high blood sugar levels can damage eyes, kidneys, nerves, and the heart, and can also lead to coma and death.

So type 1 diabetes must be treated through a daily regimen of insulin therapy.

What are the Warning Signs of Type 1 Diabetes?

The onset of type 1 diabetes happens very quickly. The following symptoms may appear suddenly and are too severe to overlook:

- Increased thirst
- Increased urination (bed-wetting may occur in children who have already been toilet trained)
- Rapid and unexplained weight loss
- Extreme hunger
- Extreme weakness or fatigue
- Unusual irritability
- Blurred vision
- Nausea, vomiting and abdominal pain
- Unpleasant breath odor
- Itchy skin

Type 1 Diabetes Treatment

Type 1 diabetes is treated by taking insulin injections or using an insulin pump or other device. This outside source of insulin now serves as the "key" -- bringing glucose to the body's cells. The challenge with taking insulin is that it's tough to know precisely how much insulin to take. The amount is based on many factors, including:

- Food
- Exercise
- Stress
- Emotions and general health

These factors change a lot throughout every day. So, deciding on what dose of insulin to take is a complicated balancing act. If you take too much insulin, then your blood sugar can drop to a dangerously low level. This is a called hypoglycemia and it can be life-threatening.

If you take too little insulin, your blood sugar can rise to a dangerously high level. Your cells are not getting the sugar, or energy, they need. This is called hyperglycemia. As mentioned above, high blood sugar levels can lead to the long-term complications and can also be life-threatening.

Today, a wide range of computerized diabetes devices are available to help people better manager their blood sugar levels while research toward a cure for diabetes moves forward.

What is Type 2 Diabetes?

The most common form of diabetes is called type 2 diabetes, or non-insulin dependent diabetes. About 90% of people with diabetes have type 2. Type 2 diabetes is also called adult onset diabetes, since it typically develops after age 35. However, a growing number of younger people are now developing type 2 diabetes.

People with type 2 diabetes are able to produce some of their own insulin. Often, it's not enough. And sometimes, the insulin will try to serve as the "key" to open the body's cells, to allow the glucose to enter. But the key won't work. The cells won't open. This is called insulin resistance. Type 2 diabetes is typically tied to people who are overweight with a sedentary lifestyle.

What are the Warning Signs of Type 2 Diabetes?

The symptoms of type 2 diabetes are similar to those of type 1 diabetes. But the onset of type 2 diabetes is usually slower and the symptoms are not as noticeable as those for type 1 diabetes. For these reasons, many people mistakenly overlook the warning signs. They also might think that the symptoms are the signs of other conditions, like aging, overworking or hot weather.

Type 2 Diabetes Treatment

Treatment for type 2 diabetes focuses on improving ways to better use the insulin the body already produces to normalize blood sugar levels. Treatment programs for type 2 diabetes focus on diet, exercise and weight loss. If blood sugar levels are still high, medications are used to help the body use its own insulin more efficiently. In some cases, insulin injections are necessary.

Chapter 2 Things You Need to Know About Meal Prepping

The Difference Between Meal Planning and Meal Prep

Meal planning and meal prep work together to ultimately serve the same purpose: to make getting weeknight dinners on the table a little easier. Meal planning is the process that asks and answers the question of "What's for dinner?" by choosing recipes that best fit your needs and schedule. Meal prep is a step in the meal planning process. It's the final critical step that puts your plan into action by readying ingredients and meals for the week ahead

The 7 Benefits of Meal Prepping

Temptation Removal

Ever been hit with hunger and have nothing on hand to eat? Yeah, that probably happens on the daily. And perhaps the only thing nearby is fast food or that leftover birthday cake your co-worker brought into the office. Meal prepping ensures you always have options that fit your dietary needs because you've planned in advance and brought your own food (or have something easy to grab from the fridge if you get a case of the munchies while watching TV). This makes sticking to your diet significantly easier.

Total Control
When you are cooking your own meals or planning what to eat in advance, you get to be a total control freak (in a good way). You gain complete calorie control and macro balance, and you limit usage of unwanted ingredients like added sugar, salt and fats. You are also ensuring you get the best-quality options and more fresh ingredients because you are selecting them yourself. In short, meal prepping is good for weight loss and for maintenance.

Hunger Manager
One of the benefits of meal preppingis that it helps you manage hunger because you are able to eat as soon as you feel hungry rather than having to wait to decide and then find a food source. Managing hunger often means you won't overeat when you finally sit down for a meal because you won't be as insanely famished.

Timesaver
When done properly, meal prepping can save quite a bit of time. Whether you simply pre-chop ingredients or cook all your meals for the week each Sunday afternoon, when you get home after a long day, you'll be thankful you don't have to take the time to go to the store or perhaps even cook. This may leave you with more time to work out, play with your kids or even enjoy a guilt-free bubble bath because you deserve it.

Money Saver
Pricing out your food in advance is another piece of the meal-prep equation, which means your portion control now has cost control. You are likely saving money because you aren't ordering out every lunch and/or dinner and can choose your meal-prep recipes based on sales at the grocery store if you wish.

Waste Eliminator
This goes hand in hand with saving money: Once you have a meal-prep routine established, you'll know exactly how much of each ingredient you need, which also cuts down on food waste. You'll never again have to witness your fruits and veggies wither away in the crisper drawer while you call for takeout.

Stress Remover
Have you ever noticed how dieting, especially cutting calories, can cause you to think about food all.day.long.? Not to mention, your willpower gets drained much faster and you are more likely to go off your plan when you're tired or "not in the mood" to make healthier choices. One of the most important benefits of meal prepping is that it can help reduce the stress that comes with trying to eat healthier. Solving all your food decisions in advance really frees up some of your willpower and mental stress, helping you reach your goals faster and with more ease.

10 Tips for Easy Meal Prep

Start small.
Identify and tackle your weak spots first — the meals or snacks that need the most attention. For example, if you're eating out every night, then start with dinner. If you can't figure out how to fit in a proper breakfast after your fasted morning workout, start with your postworkout meal.

Keep it simple, stupid.
Variety is the spice of life, but build that in over time. Initially, it's more important to keep meal prepmanageable so you're more likely to stick with it. Pick just a few proteins, veggies and starches to cook. Go ahead and pack some items raw if you don't want to cook everything. Buy pre-chopped veggies, bagged salads, and frozen and canned produce to minimize prep time. Take baby steps so you don't feel overwhelmed. That being said, if you are a proficient cook, adding culinary flair to your meal prep will stave off potential boredom. In that case, don't be afraid to add some more advanced recipes to your meal-prep rotation.

Make a list, check it twice.
The most surprising meal-prep help? It's not a sous chef, it's a grocery list! Write it down ahead of time, and remember to include items like spices, marinades and any prep tools you might need, like tinfoil or a big baking sheet. The initial trip may be a big investment, but once you've gotten into a routine, you'll be able to beeline to the exact ingredients you need for your staple recipes. You may need to grab some fresh fruits and veggies midweek, but you'll still save plenty of time by stocking up in advance.

Make cleanup a breeze.
Simplify the prep and cleanup processes with big freezer bags, tinfoil and cooking spray. You can toss ingredients in a bag with seasoning or marinade to quickly and evenly coat them. After roasting or baking, you can toss the tinfoil and your pan will immediately be ready for another round. Also, wash dishes as you go so you aren't overwhelmed by a big pile in the sink.

Practice those knife skills.
Chop ingredients in advance and in similarly sized pieces so they all cook evenly. Keep in mind that they may need to cook separately, though: Compared to sturdy veggies like broccoli, cauliflower and carrots, softer veggies like zucchini or yellow squash will cook much faster at the same temperature. If you put them all together on the same pan, you may end up with a mixture of burned and undercooked veggies.

Order matters.
Save even more time by multitasking. Start your baking or roasting first, then move to stove-top cooking and microwaving. You can roast your sturdy, starchy veggies while you saute some chicken breast. Potatoes bake quickly in the microwave, and you can find bags of steamable veggies at most grocers.

Frozen is fine.
Frozen fruits and vegetables are at least as nutritious as the fresh versions. Because they're frozen immediately after being taken off the vine, they may have even better nutrient integrity than the fresh alternative, which have spent days or weeks in transit before arriving at the grocery store. Plus, they last a lot longer. Fruits and vegetables with a low water content freeze well, so you can always chop and create your own blends that are identical to the store brand. Simply toss a mixture of broccoli, cauliflower and carrots into a freezer bag, press all the air out and throw it in the freezer. You're ready for the next meal prep!

Prevent waste.
If you are using a buffet-style meal prep, weigh your bulk items before and after cooking to determine your yield. You'll then know exactly how much you need to buy on your next shopping trip. This prevents both food waste and an inconvenient midweek emergency shopping trip.

Freezing and reheating.
You can freeze and reheat meals that you've already cooked, and in most cases, this doesn't affect the taste or texture. However, there are some exceptions: Fully cooked potatoes, zucchini and leafy greens do not rejuvenate after a freeze-thaw cycle. Experiment with just a small batch first if you want to test your recipe.

Food safety.
In general, cooked food is safe for three to four days in the fridge. If you won't eat all of it within that time frame, you can freeze it for a couple of months. Use an erasable marker on your prepped containers and a permanent marker on anything that goes into the freezer in order to document the date it was prepared or frozen. Also, when you're done prepping, food should be refrigerated within two hours of preparation but ideally immediately.

Breakfast Recipes

Bell Pepper Pancakes

Cooking Time: 8 minutes
Serves: 2

Ingredients:
- ½ cup chickpea flour
- ¼ teaspoon baking powder
- Pinch of sea salt
- Pinch of red pepper flakes, crushed
- ½ cup plus 2 tablespoons filtered water
- ¼ cup green bell peppers, seeded and chopped finely
- ¼ cup scallion, chopped finely
- 2 teaspoons olive oil

Directions:
1. In a bowl, mix together flour, baking powder, salt and red pepper flakes.
2. Add the water and mix until well combined. Fold in bell pepper and scallion.
3. In a large frying pan, heat the oil over low heat.
4. Add half of the mixture and cook for about 1-2 minutes per side.
5. Repeat with the remaining mixture. Serve warm.

Sweet Potato Waffles

Cooking Time: 20 minutes
Serves: 2

Ingredients:
- 1 medium sweet potato, peeled, grated and squeezed
- 1 teaspoon fresh thyme, minced
- 1 teaspoon fresh rosemary, minced
- 1/8 teaspoon red pepper flakes, crushed
- Salt and ground black pepper, as required

Directions:
1. Preheat the waffle iron and then grease it.
2. In a large bowl, add all ingredients and mix till well combined.
3. Place half of the sweet potato mixture into preheated waffle iron and cook for about 8-10 minutes or until golden brown.
4. Repeat with the remaining mixture. Serve warm.

Quinoa Bread

Cooking Time: 1½ hours
Serves: 12

Ingredients:
- 1¾ cups uncooked quinoa, rinsed, soaked overnight and drained
- ¼ cup chia seeds, soaked in ½ cup of water overnight
- ½ teaspoon bicarbonate soda
- Pinch of sea salt
- ½ cup filtered water
- ¼ cup olive oil, melted
- 1 tablespoon fresh lemon juice

Directions:
1. Preheat the oven to 320 degrees F. Line a loaf pan with a parchment paper.
2. In a food processor, add all the ingredients and pulse for about 3 minutes.
3. Transfer the mixture into prepared loaf pan evenly.
4. Bake for about 1½ hours or until a wooden skewer inserted in the center of loaf comes out clean.
5. Remove the pan from oven and place onto a wire rack to cool for about 10-15 minutes.
6. Carefully, remove the bread from the loaf pan and place onto the wire rack to cool completely before slicing.
7. With a sharp knife, cut the bread loaf into desired sized slices and serve.

Tofu Scramble

Cooking Time: 15 minutes
Serves: 2

Ingredients:
- ½ tablespoon olive oil
- 1 small onion, chopped finely
- 1 small red bell pepper, seeded and chopped finely
- 1 cup cherry tomatoes, chopped finely
- 1½ cups firm tofu, pressed and crumbled
- Pinch of ground turmeric
- Pinch of cayenne pepper
- 1 tablespoon fresh parsley, chopped

Directions:
1. In a skillet, heat the oil over medium heat and sauté the onion and bell pepper for about 4-5 minute.
2. Add the tomatoes and cook for about 1-2 minutes.
3. Add the tofu, turmeric and cayenne pepper and cook for about 6-8 minutes.
4. Garnish with parsley and serve.

Apple Omelet

Cooking Time: 10 minutes

Serves: 3

Ingredients:

- 4 teaspoons olive oil, divided
- 2 small green apples, cored and sliced thinly
- ¼ teaspoon ground cinnamon
- Pinch of ground cloves
- Pinch of ground nutmeg
- 4 large eggs
- ¼ teaspoon organic vanilla extract
- Pinch of salt

Directions:

1. In a large nonstick frying pan, heat 1 teaspoon of oil over medium-low heat.
2. Place the apple slices and sprinkle with spices.
3. Cook for about 4-5 minutes, flipping once halfway through.
4. Meanwhile, in a bowl, add the eggs, vanilla extract and salt and beat until fluffy.
5. Add the remaining oil in the pan and let it heat completely.
6. Place the egg mixture over apple slices evenly and cook for about 3-5 minutes or until desired doneness.
7. Carefully, turn the pan over a serving plate and immediately, fold the omelet.
8. Serve immediately.

Veggie Frittata

Cooking Time: 25 minutes

Serves: 6

Ingredients:

- 1 tablespoon olive oil
- 1 large sweet potato, peeled and cut into thin slices
- 1 yellow squash, sliced
- 1 zucchini, sliced
- ½ of red bell pepper, seeded and sliced
- ½ of yellow bell pepper, seeded and sliced
- 8 eggs
- Salt and ground black pepper, as required
- 2 tablespoons fresh cilantro, chopped finely

Directions:

1. Preheat the oven to broiler.
2. In a large oven proof skillet, heat the oil over medium-low heat and cook the sweet potato for about 6-7 minutes.
3. Add the yellow squash, zucchini and bell peppers and cook for about 3-4 minutes.
4. Meanwhile, in a bowl, add the eggs, salt and black pepper and beat until well combined.
5. Pour egg mixture over vegetables mixture evenly.
6. Immediately, reduce the heat to low and cook for about 8-10 minutes or until just done.
7. Transfer the skillet in the oven and broil for about 3-4 minutes or until top becomes golden brown.
8. With a sharp knife, cut the frittata in desired size slices and serve with the garnishing of cilantro.

Chicken & Sweet Potato Hash

Cooking Time: 35 minutes

Serves: 8

Ingredients:

- 2 tablespoons olive oil, divided
- 1½ pounds boneless, skinless chicken breasts, cubed
- Salt and ground black pepper, as required
- 2 celery stalks, chopped
- 1 medium white onion, chopped
- 4 garlic cloves, minced
- 1 tablespoon fresh oregano, chopped
- 1 tablespoon fresh thyme, chopped
- 2 large sweet potatoes, peeled and cubed
- 1 cup low-sodium chicken broth
- 1 cup scallion, chopped
- 2 tablespoons fresh lime juice

Directions:

1. In a large skillet, heat 1 tablespoon of oil over medium heat and cook the chicken with a little salt and black pepper for about 4-5 minutes.
2. Transfer the chicken into a bowl.
3. In the same skillet, heat the remaining oil over medium heat and sauté celery and onion for about 3-4 minutes.
4. Add the garlic and herbs and sauté for about 1 minute.
5. Add the sweet potato and cook for about 8-10 minutes.
6. Add the broth and cook for about 8-10 minutes.
7. Add the cooked chicken and scallion and cook for about 5 minutes.
8. Stir in lemon juice, salt and serve.

MINI VEGGIE QUICHE

Cooking Time: 15 mins

Serves: 12 mini quiches

Ingredients:

- 9 eggs
- 8 ounces of chopped spinach
- 1 small red pepper, chopped
- 1 cup of milk
- 1 cup of shredded cheddar
- 1/2 teaspoon of salt
- 1 small red onion, chopped
- Butter

Directions:
1. In a large sauté pan, add a tablespoon of butter and melt it over a medium low heat.
2. Add in the onions and cook until just translucent, for about 2 minutes.
3. Add in the spinach and cook until it's wilted.
4. Add the red peppers and more butter if needed.
5. Sauté for about 1 minute and set it aside.
6. Grease a muffin pan that holds 12 muffins.
7. Divide the sautéed veggies between the tins.
8. In a large mixing bowl, crack the 9 eggs and add in the milk and salt. Whisk together.
9. Divide half of the cheddar cheese between the muffin tins.
10. Then divide the egg mixture.
11. Bake for about 10 minutes at 375 degrees F.
12. Remove from heat and divide the rest of the cheddar, topping the quiches.
13. Place it back into the oven and bake until the eggs are set. You can use toothpick to check.
14. Remove from heat and let it cool.
15. Serve and enjoy.

SHAKSHUKA

Cooking Time: 20 mins

Serves: 6 servings

Ingredients:

- 4 garlic cloves, finely chopped
- 2 teaspoons of paprika
- 1 teaspoon of cumin
- 1 medium onion, diced
- 1 red bell pepper, deseeded and diced
- 1/4 teaspoon of chili powder
- 1 28-ounces can of whole peeled tomatoes
- 1 small bunch of fresh cilantro, chopped
- 1 small bunch of fresh parsley, chopped
- 6 large eggs
- salt and pepper, to taste

Directions:

1. In a large sauté pan, heat olive oil on medium heat.
2. Add the chopped onion and bell pepper. Then cook until the onion becomes translucent, for about 5 minutes.
3. Add spices and garlic, then cook for another minute.
4. Pour the juice and can of tomatoes into the pan, then use a large spoon to break down the tomatoes.
5. Season with pepper and salt and bring the sauce to a simmer.
6. Make small wells in the sauce using a large spoon and crack the eggs into each well.
7. Cover the pan and cook until the eggs are done to your liking, for about 5 to 8 minutes.
8. Garnish with parsley and chopped cilantro.
9. Serve and enjoy.

HEALTHY GRANOLA

Cooking Time: 25 mins
Serves: 6 cups

Ingredients:

- 2 teaspoons of ground cinnamon
- 3/4 teaspoon of fine sea salt
- 1/2 cup of melted coconut oil
- 4 cups of old-fashioned oats
- 2/3 cup of unsweetened coconut flakes (or 1/2 cup of shredded coconut)
- 1 cup of slivered almonds (or your preferred kind of seeds/nuts)
- 1/4 cup of chia seeds (optional)
- 1/3 cup of maple syrup
- 2 teaspoons of vanilla extract
- 1/2 cup of chopped dried fruit or semisweet chocolate chips (optional)

Directions:

1. Heat oven to 350 degrees F.
2. Use parchment paper to line a large baking sheet and set it aside.
3. Stir together almonds, oats, cinnamon and sea salt in a large mixing bowl until evenly combined.
4. Stir together the maple syrup, melted coconut oil and vanilla extract in a separate measuring cup until well combined.
5. Pour the coconut oil mixture into the oats mixture.
6. Stir until evenly combined.
7. Spread the granola out on the prepared baking sheet.
8. Bake, stirring once halfway through, for about 20 minutes.
9. Remove from the oven and add the coconut and stir the mixture well.
10. Bake until the granola is lightly golden and toasted, for about 5 more minutes.
11. Remove from the oven, then transfer to a wire baking rack.
12. Let it cool till the granola reaches room temp.
13. Then stir in the chocolate chips, dried fruit or any other optional add-ins you might prefer.
14. Serve immediately or store in an airtight container at room temp.
15. Enjoy.

CINNAMON OATMEAL MUFFINS WITH APPLE

Cooking Time: 15 mins
Serves: 12 muffins

Ingredients:

Topping:
- 1 tablespoon of melted butter
- 1/4 cup of quick-cooking oats
- 1 tablespoon of brown sugar
- 1/4 teaspoon of ground cinnamon

Muffins:
- 1 - 1/2 teaspoons of ground cinnamon
- 1 teaspoon of baking powder
- 1 egg, lightly beaten
- 1 teaspoon of vanilla extract
- 1/2 teaspoon of baking soda
- 1/2 teaspoon of salt
- 1 1/2 cups of quick-cooking oats
- 1 1/4 cups of all-purpose flour
- 2 tablespoons of all-purpose flour
- 1/2 cup of brown sugar
- 1/2 cup of unsweetened applesauce
- 1/2 cup of milk
- 1/4 cup of vegetable oil
- 1 apple chopped, peeled and cored

Directions:
1. Preheat oven to 400 degrees F.
2. Grease a 12-cup muffin tin and line with paper liners.
3. Stir 1 tablespoon of brown sugar, 1/4 cup of oats, 1/4 teaspoon of cinnamon and melted butter together in a small bowl. Set it aside.
4. Whisk 1/2 cup of brown sugar, 1 1/2 cups of oats, flour, baking powder, 1 1/2 teaspoons of cinnamon, salt and baking soda together in a large bowl.
5. Stir milk, applesauce, oil, egg and vanilla extract together in a bowl.
6. Stir applesauce mixture into flour mixture just until all ingredients are moistened.
7. Stir in the apple and spoon of apple mixture into prepared muffins cups, for about 2/3 full, sprinkle oat and top mixture evenly over each muffin.
8. Bake in the preheated oven, for about 15 minutes until a toothpick inserted near the center comes out clean.
9. Serve and enjoy.

VEGGIE OMELET

Cooking Time: 15 mins
Serves: 2 servings

Ingredients:
- 4 eggs
- 2 tablespoons of milk
- 3/4 teaspoon of salt
- 2 tablespoons of butter
- 1 small onion, chopped
- 1 green bell pepper, chopped
- 1/8 teaspoon of freshly ground black pepper
- 2 ounces of shredded Swiss cheese

Directions:
1. In a medium skillet, melt 1 tablespoon of butter over medium heat.
2. Place bell pepper and onion inside the skillet.
3. Cook until vegetables are just tender, for about 5 minutes, stirring occasionally.
4. Beat the eggs with 1/2 teaspoon of salt and pepper with milk while the vegetables are cooking.
5. In a small bowl, shred the cheese and set it aside.
6. Remove the vegetables from the heat.
7. Transfer them into a separate bowl and sprinkle the rest of the salt over them.
8. Melt the rest of the butter over medium heat.
9. Coat the skillet with the butter.
10. Add the egg mixture while the butter is bubbly and cook the egg until the eggs begin to set on the bottom of the pan, for about 2 minutes.
11. Lift the edges of the omelet gently using a spatula to let the uncooked part of the eggs flows to the edges and cook.
12. Continue cooking until the center of the omelet starts to look dry, for about 3 minutes.
13. Sprinkle the cheese over the omelet.
14. Spoon the vegetable mixture into the center of the omelet.
15. Using a spatula gently fold one edge of the omelet, over the vegetables,
16. Let the omelet cook until the cheese melts to your desired consistency, for about 2 minutes.
17. Slide the omelet out of the skillet and place on a plate.
18. Cut into half, serve and enjoy.

Spinach Scramble

Cooking Time: 15 minutes

Serves: 2

Ingredients:

- ¼ cup liquid egg substitute
- ¼ cup skim milk
- Salt and pepper to taste
- 2 tablespoons crumbled bacon
- 13 ½ oz. canned spinach, drained
- Cooking spray

Directions:

1. Mix all the ingredients in a large bowl.
2. Pour the mixture on a pan greased with oil, placed over medium heat.
3. Stir until fully cooked.
4. Calories: 70 calories, Carbohydrates: 5 g, Protein: 8 g, Fat: 2 g, Saturated Fat: 1 g, Sodium: 700 mg, Fiber: 2 g

Breakfast Parfait

Cooking Time: 0 minute

Serves: 2

Ingredients:

- 4 oz. unsweetened applesauce
- 6 oz. non-fat and sugar-free vanilla yogurt
- ¼ teaspoon pumpkin pie spice
- ¼ teaspoon honey
- 1 cup low-fat granola

Directions:

1. Mix all the ingredients except the granola in a bowl.
2. Layer the mixture with the granola in a cup.
3. Refrigerate before serving.

Asparagus & Cheese Omelet

Cooking Time: 10 minutes

Serves: 2

Ingredients:

- Cooking spray
- 4 spears asparagus, sliced
- Pepper to taste
- 3 egg whites
- ½ teaspoon olive oil
- 1 oz. spreadable cheese, sliced
- 1 teaspoon parsley, chopped

Directions:

1. Spray oil on your pan.
2. Cook asparagus on the pan over medium high heat for 5 to 7 minutes.
3. Wrap with foil and set aside.
4. In a bowl, mix pepper and egg whites.
5. Add olive oil to the pan.
6. Add the egg whites.
7. When you start to see the sides forming, add the asparagus and cheese on top.
8. Use a spatula to lift and fold the egg.
9. Sprinkle parsley on top before serving.

Lunch Recipes

TORTILLA CHICKEN SOUP

Cooking Time: 30 mins
Serves: 8 servings

Ingredients:
- 1 cup of corn, drained if canned
- 2 chicken breasts boneless, skinless
- 1/4 cup of cilantro chopped
- 1 lime juiced
- 1 sliced avocado
- 1 tablespoon of olive oil
- 1 chopped onion
- 3 large cloves garlic, minced
- 1 jalapeño deseeded and diced
- 1 teaspoon of ground cumin
- 1 teaspoon of chili powder
- 14.5 ounces of crushed tomatoes
- 1 can diced tomatoes with chilies
- 3 cups of chicken broth
- 14.5 ounce can black beans, drained and rinsed
- Crispy Tortilla Strips
- 1/4 cup of olive oil
- salt
- 6 6-inches corn tortillas cut into 1/4-inch strips

Directions:
1. Over medium high heat, heat 1/4 cup of olive oil in a small pan.
2. Add tortilla strips into small batches and then fry till crisp.
3. Drain and add sprinkle salt.
4. In a large pot over medium heat, heat olive oil and add garlic, onion, jalapeno and onion, then cook until softened.
5. Add the rest of the ingredients and simmer until chicken is cooked through, for about 20 minutes.
6. Remove chicken and shred it.
7. Add it back to the pot and then simmer for just 3 mins.
8. Spoon your soup into bowls.
9. Top with lime wedges, tortilla strips and sliced avocado.
10. Serve and enjoy.

CHICKEN BROCCOLI SALAD

Cooking Time: 0 mins

Serves: 10 servings

Ingredients:

- 1/4 cup of apple cider vinegar
- 1/4 cup of white sugar
- 1/4 cup of crumbled cooked bacon
- 8 cups of broccoli florets
- 3 cooked skinless, boneless chicken breast halves, cubed
- 1 cup of chopped walnuts
- 6 green onions, chopped
- 1 cup of mayonnaise

Directions:

1. Combine chicken, broccoli, walnuts and green onions in a large bowl.
2. Whisk together vinegar, mayonnaise and sugar in a bowl until it's well blended.
3. Pour mayonnaise dressing over broccoli mixture and toss to coat.
4. Cover and refrigerate till chilled if you feel like.
5. To serve: sprinkle with crumbled bacon.
6. Serve and enjoy.

BLACK BEAN SALAD

Cooking Time: 0 mins

Serves: 6 servings

Ingredients:

- 1 avocado, deseeded, peeled and cut into chunks
- 1/2 to 1 teaspoon of sugar (to taste)
- Salt and pepper to taste
- 1/2 cup of chopped fresh cilantro
- 1 1/2 cups of freshly cooked black beans (or 1 (15 ounces) can of black beans, drained and rinsed)
- 1 1/2 cups of frozen corn, defrosted (or fresh corn, drained, parboiled and cooled, or cooled and grilled)
- 1/2 cup of shallots or chopped green onions (including onion greens)
- 2 tablespoons of lime juice (about the juice from one lime)
- 1 tablespoon of extra virgin olive oil
- 1/2 fresh jalapeño pepper, minced and deseeded, or 1/2 pickled jalapeño pepper, minced (not seeded)
- 3 fresh plum tomatoes, deseeded and chopped and/or 1 red bell pepper, chopped and deseeded

Directions:

1. Combine the corn, black beans, minced jalapenos, chopped green onions, chopped tomatoes or red bell pepper, olive oil and lime juice in a large bowl.
2. Fold in the chopped avocado gently.
3. Add pepper and salt to taste.
4. Sprinkle with sugar to taste (sugar that is enough to balance the acidity from the lime juice).
5. Chill before serving.
6. Add the chopped fresh cilantro.
7. Serve and enjoy.

KALE SALAD WITH LEMON DRESSING

Cooking Time: 0 mins

Serves: 4 servings

Ingredients:

Lemon Dressing

- 1 minced garlic clove
- 1 teaspoon of dried oregano
- 1/2 cup of extra virgin olive oil
- 1/4 cup of lemon juice
- Salt and pepper to taste

Kale Salad

- 1/2 red onion thinly sliced
- 1/2 cup of crumbled feta cheese
- 1-pint cherry or grape tomatoes halved
- 1 large bunch of about 10 ounces (or 3-4 cups of kale leaves), finely chopped
- 1 cucumber deseeded and diced

Directions:

Making the Lemon Dressing:

1. Combine together the lemon juice, garlic, olive oil, salt, oregano and pepper in a small or medium mixing bowl.
2. Whisk until well combined.

Making the Kale Salad:

3. Add together all the chopped ingredients in a large bowl and combine.
4. Pour the dressing over the salad and mix together.
5. Sprinkle with some feta cheese just before serving.
6. You can store your dressed and prepared salad in the fridge for up to 2 days.
7. Serve and enjoy.

CARROT GINGER SOUP

Cooking Time: 30 mins

Serves: 4 servings

Ingredients:

- 1 tablespoon of apple cider vinegar
- 3 to 4 cups of vegetable broth
- Sea salt and fresh black pepper
- 1 tablespoon of extra-virgin olive oil
- 1 cup of chopped yellow onions
- 3 garlic cloves, smashed
- 2 heaping cups of chopped carrots
- 1 - 1/2 teaspoons of grated fresh ginger
- 1 teaspoon of maple syrup, or to taste (optional)
- coconut milk for garnish, optional
- dollops of pesto, optional

Directions:

1. In a large pot, heat the olive oil over medium heat.
2. Add the onions and a pinch of salt and pepper.
3. Cook until softened, stirring occasionally, for about 8 minutes.
4. Add the smashed garlic cloves and the chopped carrots into the pot.
5. Cook for another 8 minutes, stirring occasionally.
6. Stir in the ginger and add the apple cider vinegar.
7. The next thing you'll want to do is add 3 to 4 cups of broth.
8. Reduce to a simmer and cook for about 30 minutes, until the carrots are soft.
9. Let it cool slightly and transfer into a blender.
10. Blend until smooth.
11. Taste and adjust seasonings.
12. Add maple syrup if you feel like.
13. Serve with a dollop of pesto or drizzle of coconut milk.
14. Enjoy.

SHRIMP SALAD

Cooking Time: 0 mins

Serves: 2 servings

Ingredients:

For the Salad:

- Freshly ground black pepper
- 1/4 finely chopped red onion
- 1 finely chopped stalk celery
- 1 pound of shrimp, deveined and peeled
- 1 tablespoon of extra-virgin olive oil
- Kosher salt
- 2 tablespoons of freshly chopped dill
- Toasted bread or butterhead or romaine lettuce, for serving

For the Dressing:

- 1/2 cup of mayonnaise
- Juice and zest of 1 lemon
- 1 teaspoon of Dijon mustard

Directions:

1. Preheat oven to 400 degrees F.
2. Toss shrimp with oil on a large baking sheet.
3. Season with pepper and salt.
4. Bake for about 5 minutes, until shrimp are completely opaque.
5. Whisk together mayonnaise, zest, lemon juice and Dijon in a large bowl.
6. Season with pepper and salt.
7. Add your cooked shrimp, celery, red onion and dill to bowl.
8. Then toss until well combined.
9. Serve over lettuce and enjoy.

CRISPY TOFU

Cooking Time: 30 mins

Serves: 4 servings

Ingredients:

- 1/4 teaspoon of garlic powder
- 1/4 teaspoon of pure maple syrup
- 1/4 teaspoon of rice wine vinegar
- 1 tablespoon of toasted sesame oil, or your favorite oil
- 1 (14 ounces) container extra firm tofu, pressed and patted dry for at least 15 minutes
- 1 teaspoon of soy sauce or tamari
- 2 teaspoons of corn starch or arrowroot powder

Directions:

1. Preheat oven to 400 degrees F.
2. Whisk together tamari or soy sauce, sesame oil, maple syrup, garlic powder and vinegar in a medium sized bowl.
3. Cut the press tofu into bite sized pieces.
4. Place the pieces into the oil mixture.
5. Stir the tofu using a spoon or spatula, making sure it's completely coated.
6. Sprinkle 1 teaspoon of the arrowroot powder over it and mix well till all of the tofu is coated.
7. Sprinkle the rest of the arrowroot powder and mix carefully just until you can't see the dry white powder anymore.
8. Using parchment paper or nonstick to line a large baking sheet.
9. Pour the tofu onto baking sheet and arrange it so that the pieces won't be touching each other.
10. Bake tofu until crispy and golden, for about 25 minutes, stirring 2 to 3 times during the baking.
11. Let the tofu sit for some minutes to crisp even more before enjoying.
12. Serve and enjoy.

SPINACH SOUP WITH PESTO & CHICKEN

Cooking Time: 20 mins
Serves: 5 servings

Ingredients:
- 1 large clove garlic, minced
- 1/8 cup of lightly packed fresh basil leaves
- Freshly ground pepper to taste
- 5 cups of reduced-sodium chicken broth
- 1 1/2 teaspoons of dried marjoram
- 6 ounces of baby spinach, coarsely chopped
- 2 teaspoons with 1 tablespoon of extra-virgin olive oil, divided
- 1/2 cup of carrot or diced red bell pepper
- 1 large boneless, skinless chicken breast (about 8 ounces), cut into quarters
- 1 15-ounces can of cannellini beans or great northern beans, rinsed
- 1/4 cup of grated Parmesan cheese
- 3/4 cup of plain or herbed multigrain croutons for garnish (optional)

Directions:
1. In a large saucepan, heat 2 tablespoons of oil over medium high heat.
2. Add carrot or bell pepper with chicken together.
3. Cook, turning the chicken and stirring occasionally, for about 3 minutes, until the chicken begins to brown.
4. Add garlic and cook, stirring, for another 1 minute.
5. Stir in marjoram and broth.
6. Bring to a boil over high heat and reduce the heat.
7. Simmer, stirring occasionally, for about 5 minutes until the chicken is cooked through. Transfer the chicken pieces to a clean cutting board to cool using a slotted spoon.
8. Add beans and spinach into the pot, then bring to a boil.
9. Cook for 5 mins to blend the flavors.
10. In a food processor, combine the parmesan, 1 tablespoon of oil, basil.
11. Process until a coarse paste forms, adding a little water and scrape down the sides. Cut the chicken into small size pieces.
12. Stir the pesto and chicken into the pot.
13. Season with pepper and heat until it's hot.
14. Garnish with croutons, if you feel like. Serve and enjoy.

Asian Cold Noodle Salad

Cooking Time: None

Serves: 1

Ingredients:

- 3 tablespoons light coconut milk
- 2 tablespoons whipped peanut butter
- 1 tablespoon water
- 1 tablespoon fresh lime juice
- ½ tablespoon soy sauce
- ¼ to ½ teaspoon sriracha sauce
- 1 ounce whole-wheat spaghetti, cooked
- ½ cup snow peas, halved
- 2 ounces cooked chicken breast, chopped
- ¼ cup diced red pepper
- 1 teaspoon fresh chopped cilantro
- 1 green onion, sliced thin

Directions:

1. Stir together the coconut milk, peanut butter, water, lime juice, soy sauce, and sriracha sauce in a small bowl.
2. Cook the spaghetti to al dente then drain and rinse under cool water.
3. Combine the cooled spaghetti, snow peas, chicken, red pepper, and cilantro in a bowl.
4. Toss with the dressing until well coated then serve with sliced green onion.

Chicken Tortilla Soup

Cooking Time: 20 minutes

Serves: 6

Ingredients:

- 1 tablespoon olive oil
- ½ small yellow onion, diced
- 3 cloves minced garlic
- 2 cups fat-free chicken broth
- 1 (15-ounce) can black beans, rinsed and drained
- 1 cup crushed tomatoes
- 2 tablespoons tomato paste
- 1 teaspoon ground cumin
- ½ teaspoon paprika
- Salt and pepper
- 8 ounces cooked chicken breast, shredded
- 1 tablespoon fresh lime juice
- 1 tablespoon fresh chopped cilantro
- 1 medium diced avocado, optional

Directions:

1. Heat the oil in a large saucepan over medium heat.
2. Add the onion and sauté for 3 minutes then stir in the garlic and cook 1 minute more.
3. Pour in the chicken broth, beans, tomatoes, tomato paste, cumin, and paprika.
4. Bring to a light boil then simmer for 10 minutes.
5. Season with salt and pepper then stir in the cooked chicken.
6. Cook until the chicken is heated through then remove from heat.
7. Stir in the lime juice and cilantro then adjust seasoning to taste.
8. Serve hot with diced avocado.

Dinner Recipes

FRENCH LENTILS

Cooking Time: 25 mins

Serves: 4 servings

Ingredients:

- 2 1/4 cups of French lentils
- 3 tablespoons of olive or vegetable oil
- 1 teaspoon of dried or fresh thyme
- 3 bay leaves
- 1 tablespoon of kosher salt
- 1 onion, peeled and finely chopped
- 2 cloves garlic, peeled and finely chopped
- 1 carrot, peeled and finely chopped

Directions:

1. Place a large saucepan over a medium heat and add oil.
2. Add chopped vegetables when hot and sauté for about 5 to 10 minutes, until softened.
3. Add lentils, 6 cups of water, thyme, salt and bay leaves.
4. Bring to a boil and reduce to a fast simmer.
5. Simmer for 20 to 25 minutes until they are tender and have absorbed most of the water.
6. Drain any excess water after lentils have cooked, if necessary.
7. Serve immediately and enjoy.

CHICKEN FAJITAS

Cooking Time: 15 mins

Serves: 4 servings

Ingredients:

- 2 teaspoons of fajita seasoning
- 1 green bell pepper, cut into strips
- 1 red bell pepper, cut into strips
- 1 clove garlic, minced
- 1 cup of sliced onion
- 2 boneless, skinless chicken breasts, cut into strips
- 4 low-carb whole wheat tortillas, warmed

Directions:

1. Cooking spray to coat a large skillet.
2. Cook garlic, bell peppers and onion over medium heat until tender, for about 6 to 8 minutes, stirring occasionally.
3. Remove to a plate.
4. Add chicken and fajita seasoning; cook until no longer pink in center, for about 5 minutes.
5. Return vegetables to skillet and cook until heated through, for about 2 to 4 more minutes.
6. Divide fajita mixture evenly onto tortillas.
7. Serve immediately and enjoy.

VEGGIE RICE

Cooking Time: 20 mins

Serves: 4 servings

Ingredients:

- 4 tablespoons of oil
- 2 cups of water
- 1 cup of basmati rice
- 1 small onion finely chopped
- 1/2 cup of frozen veggies. You can use a mix of corn, carrots, peas and green beans
- Salt and pepper to taste.

Directions:

1. Heat the oil in a pot and fry the onion till translucent.
2. Add the pepper, frozen veggies, salt and cook for 5 minutes.
3. Add the water, and use lid to cover the pot.
4. Bring water to a boil and then add the rice.
5. Cook on medium high heat till rice is almost cooked and most of the water has evaporated.
6. Lower the heat and cover the rice.
7. Let the rice steam until it's completely cooked, for about 5 minutes.
8. Remove from heat and use fork to fluff the rice.
9. Serve immediately.
10. Enjoy.

GRILLED TUNA KEBABS

Cooking Time: 0 mins

Serves: 4 servings

Ingredients:

- 3 tablespoons of fresh lime juice (from 2 limes)
- freshly ground pepper and coarse salt.
- 1 1/2 pounds of sushi-grade yellowfin tuna (cut into 1 1/2-inch cubes)
- 1/4 cup plus 2 tablespoons of extra-virgin olive oil
- 3 tablespoons of chopped fresh cilantro

Directions:

1. Heat a grill pan over medium heat.
2. Toss tuna with 1 tablespoon of oil.
3. Thread tuna onto 4 kebabs.
4. Combine lime juice, cilantro and 1/4 cup of oil.
5. Season with pepper and salt.
6. Reserve about 3 tablespoons.
7. Brush pan with the remaining tablespoon of oil.
8. Grill tuna, turning kebabs and brushing tuna occasionally with lime sauce, for about 2 minutes per side for rare or to desired doneness.
9. Transfer kebabs to a serving plate.
10. Brush with reserved lime sauce.
11. Serve immediately and enjoy.

SPICY TURKEY TACOS

Cooking Time: 0 mins

Serves: 4 servings

Ingredients:

- 1/2 teaspoon of ground cumin
- 2 cups of shredded lettuce
- 8 taco shells
- 1/2 teaspoon of dried oregano
- 1/2 teaspoon of paprika
- 1/2 teaspoon of ground cinnamon
- 1 pound of extra-lean ground turkey
- 1 small red onion, finely chopped
- 1 cup of salsa
- 1/2 cup of shredded pepper jack cheese
- 1/4 cup of fat-free sour cream
- Cubed avocado and extra salsa, optional

Directions:

1. Heat taco shells just according to the directions in the package.
2. Cook turkey and onion in a large nonstick skillet over medium heat until the meat is no longer pink.
3. Stir in spices and salsa.
4. Heat through and serve immediately.
5. Fill each of the taco shell with 1/3 cup of turkey mixture if you want to serve.
6. Serve with cheese, lettuce or sour cream if you feel like.
7. Enjoy.

LIME QUINOA WITH CILANTRO

Cooking Time: 25 mins

Serves: 6 servings

Ingredients:

- 1 mango, diced and peeled
- 1 diced jalapeno pepper
- 1/4 teaspoon of salt
- 1 avocado - peeled, pitted, and diced
- 1 1/2 tablespoons of lime juice
- 2 tablespoons of chopped fresh cilantro
- 1 tablespoon of olive oil
- 2 cloves garlic, minced
- 1/2 red onion, diced
- 1 cup of quinoa, rinsed and drained
- 1 1/2 cups of low-sodium chicken broth
- 1 cup of corn

Directions:

1. In a saucepan, heat olive oil over medium heat
2. Cook and stir garlic until fragrant for about 1 minute.
3. Add jalapeno pepper, onion and salt.
4. Cook and stir for about 5 to 10 minutes, until onion is tender.
5. Add quinoa and cook for 2 minutes until slightly browned.
6. Pour in the chicken broth, then bring to a boil.
7. Reduce heat to low and simmer for about 15 minutes until broth is absorbed.
8. Stir mango, corn, lime juice, avocado and cilantro into the quinoa mixture.
9. Serve immediately and enjoy.

POTATOES WITH ROASTED VEGGIES

Cooking Time: 40 mins

Serves: 12 servings

Ingredients:

- 1 red onion, quartered
- 1 tablespoon of chopped fresh thyme
- 2 tablespoons of chopped fresh rosemary
- 1/4 cup of olive oil
- 2 tablespoons of balsamic vinegar
- 1 small butternut squash, cubed
- 2 red bell peppers, deseeded and diced
- 1 sweet potato, peeled and cubed
- 3 Yukon Gold potatoes, cubed
- salt and freshly ground black pepper

Directions:

1. Preheat oven to 475 degrees F.
2. Combine the red bell peppers, squash, Yukon gold potatoes and sweet potato in a large bowl.
3. Separate the red onion quarters into pieces, then add them into the mixture.
4. Stir together rosemary, thyme, vinegar, salt, olive oil, pepper and salt in a small bowl.
5. Toss with vegetables till they're coated.
6. Spread evenly on a large roasting pan.
7. Roast for about 35 minutes in the preheated oven, until vegetables are cooked through and browned, turn the vegetables every 10 minutes.
8. Serve and enjoy.

MUSHROOM STROGANOFF

Cooking Time: 20 mins
Serves: 4 servings

Ingredients:

- 3 cloves garlic, minced
- 4 teaspoons of chopped fresh thyme
- 2 1/2 tablespoons of all-purpose flour
- 2 cups of beef stock
- 2 tablespoons of chopped fresh parsley leaves
- 8 ounces of medium pasta shells
- 3 tablespoons of unsalted butter
- 1 1/2 pounds of cremini mushrooms, thinly sliced
- 2 large shallots, diced
- Kosher salt and freshly ground black pepper, to taste
- 1 1/2 teaspoons of Dijon mustard
- 3/4 cup of sour cream
- 2/3 cup of freshly grated Parmesan

Directions:

1. Cook pasta according to package instructions in a large pot of boiling salted water. Drain it well.
2. In a large skillet, melt butter over medium high heat.
3. Add shallots and mushrooms and cook, stirring occasionally, until mushrooms are browned and tender, for about 5 minutes.
4. Season with pepper and salt, to taste.
5. Stir in thyme and garlic, cook for 1 minute, until fragrant.
6. Whisk in flour cook for 1 minute, until lightly browned.
7. Whisk in beef stock and Dijon gradually and bring it to a boil.
8. Reduce heat and simmer, stirring occasionally, until slightly thickened and reduced, for about 5 minutes.
9. Stir in sour cream and pasta until heated through, for about 2 minutes.
10. Stir in Parmesan for 1 minute, until melted.
11. Stir in parsley, season with pepper and salt, to taste.
12. Serve immediately and enjoy.

Almond-Crusted Salmon

Cooking Time: 15 minutes

Serves: 4

Ingredients:

- ¼ cup almond meal
- ¼ cup whole-wheat breadcrumbs
- ¼ teaspoon ground coriander
- 1/8 teaspoon ground cumin
- 4 (6-ounce) boneless salmon fillets
- 1 tablespoon fresh lemon juice
- Salt and pepper

Directions:

1. Preheat the oven to 500°F and line a small baking dish with foil.
2. Combine the almond meal, breadcrumbs, coriander, and cumin in a small bowl.
3. Rinse the fish in cool water then pat dry and brush with lemon juice.
4. Season the fish with salt and pepper then dredge in the almond mixture on both sides.
5. Place the fish in the baking dish and bake for 15 minutes until it just flakes with a fork.

Chicken & Veggie Bowl with Brown Rice

Cooking Time: 20 minutes
Serves: 4

Ingredients:

- 1 cup instant brown rice
- ¼ cup tahini
- ¼ cup fresh lemon juice
- 2 cloves minced garlic
- ¼ teaspoon ground cumin
- Pinch salt
- 1 tablespoon olive oil
- 4 (4-ounce) chicken breast halves
- ½ medium yellow onion, sliced
- 1 cup green beans, trimmed
- 1 cup chopped broccoli
- 4 cups chopped kale

Directions:

1. Bring 1 cup water to boil in a small saucepan.
2. Stir in the brown rice and simmer for 5 minutes then cover and set aside.
3. Meanwhile, whisk together the tahini with ¼ cup water in a small bowl.
4. Stir in the lemon juice, garlic, and cumin with a pinch of salt and stir well.
5. Heat the oil in a large cast-iron skillet over medium heat.
6. Season the chicken with salt and pepper then add to the skillet.
7. Cook for 3 to 5 minutes on each side until cooked through then remove to a cutting board and cover loosely with foil.
8. Reheat the skillet and cook the onion for 2 minutes then stir in the broccoli and beans.
9. Sauté for 2 minutes then stir in the kale and sauté 2 minutes more.
10. Add 2 tablespoons of water then cover and steam for 2 minutes while you slice the chicken.
11. Build the bowls with brown rice, sliced chicken, and sautéed veggies.
12. Serve hot drizzled with the lemon tahini dressing.

Meat Recipes

Beef Salad

Cooking Time: 8 minutes

Serves: 6

Ingredients:

For Steak:

- 1½ pounds skirt steak, trimmed and cut into 4 pieces
- Salt and ground black pepper, as required

For Salad:

- 2 medium green bell pepper, seeded and sliced thinly
- 2 large tomatoes, sliced
- 1 cup onion, sliced thinly
- 8 cups mixed fresh baby greens

For Dressing:

- 2 teaspoons Dijon mustard
- 4 tablespoons balsamic vinegar
- ½ cup olive oil
- Salt and ground black pepper, as required

Directions:

1. Preheat the grill to medium-high heat. Grease the grill grate.
2. Sprinkle the beef steak with a little salt and black pepper.
3. Place the steak onto the grill and cook, covered for about 3-4 minutes per side. Transfer the steak onto a cutting board for about 10 minutes before slicing.
4. With a sharp knife, cut the beef steaks into thin slices.
5. Meanwhile, in a large bowl, mix together all salad ingredients.
6. For dressing: in another bowl, add all the ingredients and beat until well combined. Pour the dressing over salad and gently toss to coat well.
7. Divide the salad onto serving plates evenly.
8. Top each plate with the steak slices and serve.

Beef Curry

Cooking Time: 40 minutes

Serves: 6

Ingredients:

- 1 cup fat-free plain Greek yogurt
- ½ teaspoon garlic paste
- ½ teaspoon ginger paste
- ½ teaspoon ground cloves
- ½ teaspoon ground cumin
- 2 teaspoons red pepper flakes, crushed
- ¼ teaspoon ground turmeric
- Salt, as required
- 2 pounds round steak, cut into pieces
- ¼ cup olive oil
- 1 medium yellow onion, thinly sliced
- 1½ tablespoons fresh lemon juice
- ¼ cup fresh cilantro, chopped

Directions:

1. In a large bowl, add the yogurt, garlic paste, ginger paste and spices and mix well.
2. Add the steak pieces and generously coat with the yogurt mixture.
3. Set aside for at least 15 minutes.
4. In a large skillet, heat the oil over medium-high heat and sauté the onion for about 4-5 minutes.
5. Add the steak pieces with marinade and stir to combine.
6. Immediately, adjust the heat to low and simmer, covered and cook for about 25 minutes, stirring occasionally.
7. Stir in the lemon juice and simmer for about 10 more minutes.
8. Garnish with fresh cilantro and serve hot.

Beef with Barley & Veggies

Cooking Time: 1 hour 5 minutes

Serves: 2

Ingredients:

- ¾ cup filtered water
- ¼ cup pearl barley
- 2 teaspoons olive oil
- 7 ounces lean ground beef
- 1 cup fresh mushrooms, sliced
- ¾ cup onion, chopped
- 2 cups frozen green beans
- ¼ cup low-sodium beef broth
- 2 tablespoon fresh parsley, chopped

Directions:

1. In a pan, add water, barley and pinch of salt and bring to a boil over medium heat.
2. Now, reduce the heat to low and simmer, covered for about 30-40 minutes or until all the liquid is absorbed.
3. Remove from heat and set aside.
4. In a skillet, heat oil over medium-high heat and cook beef for about 8-10 minutes.
5. Add the mushroom and onion and cook f or about 6-7 minutes.
6. Add the green beans and cook for about 2-3 minutes.
7. Stir in cooked barley and broth and cook for about 3-5 minutes more.
8. Stir in the parsley and serve hot.

Beef with Broccoli

Cooking Time: 14 minutes

Serves: 4

Ingredients:

- 2 tablespoons olive oil, divided
- 2 garlic cloves, minced
- 1 pound beef sirloin steak, trimmed and sliced into thin strips
- ¼ cup low-sodium chicken broth
- 2 teaspoons fresh ginger, grated
- 1 tablespoon ground flax seeds
- ½ teaspoon red pepper flakes, crushed
- Salt and ground black pepper, as required
- 1 large carrot, peeled and sliced thinly
- 2 cups broccoli florets
- 1 medium scallion, sliced thinly

Directions:

1. In a large skillet, heat 1 tablespoon of oil over medium-high heat and sauté the garlic for about 1 minute.
2. Add the beef and cook for about 4-5 minutes or until browned.
3. With a slotted spoon, transfer the beef into a bowl.
4. Remove the excess liquid from skillet.
5. In a bowl, add the broth, ginger, flax seeds, red pepper flakes, salt and black pepper.
6. In the same skillet, heat remaining oil over medium heat.
7. Add the carrot, broccoli and ginger mixture and cook for about 3-4 minutes or until desired doneness.
8. Stir in beef and scallion and cook for about 3-4 minutes.

Pan Grilled Steak

Cooking Time: 16 minutes

Serves: 4

Ingredients:

- 8 medium garlic cloves, crushed
- 1 (2-inch) piece fresh ginger, sliced thinly
- ¼ cup olive oil
- Salt and ground black pepper, as required
- 1½ pounds flank steak, trimmed

Directions:

1. In a large sealable bag, mix together all ingredients except steak.
2. Add the steak and coat with marinade generously.
3. Seal the bag and refrigerate to marinate for about 24 hours.
4. Remove from refrigerator and keep in room temperature for about 15 minutes.
5. Discard the excess marinade from steak.
6. Heat a lightly greased grill pan over medium-high heat and cook the steak for about 6-8 minutes per side.
7. Remove from grill pan and set aside for about 10 minutes before slicing.
8. With a sharp knife cut into desired slices and serve.

Lamb Stew

Preparation Time: 15 minutes

Cooking Time: 2¼ hours

Serves: 8

Ingredients:

- 1 teaspoon ground cumin
- 1 teaspoon ground coriander
- ½ teaspoon cayenne pepper
- ½ teaspoon ground cinnamon
- 2 tablespoons olive oil
- 3 pounds lamb stew meat, trimmed and cubed
- Sea Salt and ground black pepper, as required
- 1 onion, chopped
- 2 garlic cloves, minced
- 2¼ cups low-sodium chicken broth
- 2 cups tomatoes, chopped finely
- 1 medium head cauliflower, cut into 1-inch florets

Directions:

1. Preheat the oven to 300 degrees F.
2. In a small bowl, mix together spices and set aside.
3. In a large ovenproof pan, heat oil over medium heat and cook the lamb with a little salt and black pepper for about 10 minutes or until browned from all sides. With a slotted spoon, transfer the lamb into a bowl.
4. In the same pan, add onion and sauté for about 3-4 minutes.
5. Add the garlic and spice mixture and sauté for about 1 minute.
6. Add the cooked lamb, broth and tomatoes and bring to a gentle boil.
7. Immediately, cover the pan and transfer into oven.
8. Bake for about 1½ hours.
9. Remove from oven and stir in cauliflower.
10. Bake for about 30 minutes more or until cauliflower is done completely.
11. Serve hot.

Lamb Curry

Cooking Time: 2¼ hours

Serves: 8

Ingredients:

For Spice Mixture:

- 2 teaspoons ground coriander
- 2 teaspoons ground cumin
- 1 teaspoon ground cinnamon
- ½ teaspoon ground ginger
- 1 tablespoons sweet paprika
- ½ tablespoon cayenne pepper
- 1 teaspoon red chili powder
- Salt and ground black pepper, as required

For Curry:

- 1 tablespoon olive oil
- 2 pounds boneless lamb, trimmed and cubed into 1-inch size
- 2 cups onions, chopped
- ½ cup fat-free plain Greek yogurt, whipped
- 1½ cups water

Directions:

1. For spice mixture: in a bowl, add all spices and mix well. Set aside.
2. In a large Dutch oven, heat the oil over medium-high heat and stir fry the lamb cubes for about 5 minutes.
3. Add the onion and cook for about 4-5 minutes.
4. Stir in the spice mixture and cook for about 1 minute.
5. Add the yogurt and water and bring to a boil over high heat.
6. Now, reduce the heat to low and simmer, covered for about 1-2 hours or until desired doneness of lamb.
7. Uncover and simmer for about 3-4 minutes.
8. Serve hot.

Meatballs in Tomato Gravy

Cooking Time: 30 minutes
Serves: 6

Ingredients:

For Meatballs:
- 1 pound lean ground lamb
- 1 tablespoon homemade tomato paste
- ¼ cup fresh cilantro leaves, chopped
- 1 small onion, chopped finely
- 2 garlic cloves, minced
- ½ teaspoon ground cumin
- 1/8 teaspoon salt
- Ground black pepper, as required

For Tomato Gravy:
- 3 tablespoons olive oil, divided
- 2 medium onions, chopped finely
- 2 garlic cloves, minced
- ½ tablespoon fresh ginger, minced
- 1 teaspoon dried thyme, crushed
- 1 teaspoon dried oregano, crushed
- 3 large tomatoes, chopped finely
- Ground black pepper, as required
- 1½ cups warm low-sodium chicken broth

Directions:

1. For meatballs: in a large bowl, add all the ingredients and mix until well combined.
2. Make small equal-sized balls from mixture and set aside.
3. For gravy: in a large pan, heat 1 tablespoon of oil over medium heat.
4. Add the meatballs and cook for about 4-5 minutes or until lightly browned from all sides.
5. With a slotted spoon, transfer the meatballs onto a plate.
6. In the same pan, heat the remaining oil over medium heat and sauté the onion for about 8-10 minutes.
7. Add the garlic, ginger and herbs and sauté for about 1 minute.
8. Add the tomatoes and cook for about 3-4 minutes, crushing with the back of spoon. Add the warm broth and bring to a boil.
9. Carefully, place the meatballs and cook for 5 minutes, without stirring.
10. Now, reduce the heat to low and cook partially covered for about 15-20 minutes, stirring gently 2-3 times. Serve hot.

Spiced Leg of Lamb

Cooking Time: 1 hour 40 minutes

Serves: 6

Ingredients:

For Marinade:

- 2/3 cup fat-free plain Greek yogurt
- 1 tablespoon homemade tomato puree
- 1 tablespoon fresh lemon juice
- 3-4 garlic cloves, minced
- 2 tablespoons fresh rosemary, chopped
- 2 teaspoons ground coriander
- 1 teaspoon ground cumin
- 1 teaspoon ground cinnamon
- 1 teaspoon red pepper flakes, crushed
- ¼ teaspoon sweet paprika
- Sea salt and freshly ground black pepper, as required
- 1 (4½-pound) bone-in leg of lamb

Directions:

1. In a large bowl, add yogurt, tomato puree, lemon juice, garlic, rosemary, and spices and mix until well combined.
2. Add leg of lamb and coat with marinade generously.
3. Cover and refrigerate to marinate for about 8-10 hours, flipping occasionally.
4. Remove the marinated leg of lamb from refrigerator and keep in room temperature for about 25-30 minutes before roasting.
5. Preheat the oven to 425 degree F.
6. Line a large roasting pan with a greased foil piece.
7. Arrange the leg of lamb into prepared roasting pan. Roast for 20 minutes.
8. Remove the roasting pan from oven and change the side of leg of lamb.
9. Now, Now, reduce the temperature of oven to 325 degree F.
10. Roast for 40 minutes.
11. Now loosely cover the roasting pan with a large piece of foil.
12. Roast for 40 minutes more. Remove from oven and place onto a cutting board for about 10-15 minutes before slicing.
13. With a sharp knife cut the leg of lamb in desired sized slices and serve.

Baked Lamb & Spinach

Cooking Time: 2 hours 55 minutes
Serves: 6

Ingredients:
- 2 tablespoons olive oil
- 2 pounds lamb necks, trimmed and cut into 2-inch pieces crosswise
- Salt, as required
- 2 medium onions, chopped
- 3 tablespoons fresh ginger, minced
- 4 garlic cloves, minced
- 2 tablespoons ground coriander
- 1 tablespoon ground cumin
- 1 teaspoon ground turmeric
- ¼ cup fat-free plain Greek yogurt
- ½ cup tomatoes, chopped
- 2 cups boiling water
- 30 ounces frozen spinach, thawed and squeezed
- 1½ tablespoons garam masala
- 1 tablespoon fresh lemon juice
- Ground black pepper, as required

Directions:
1. Preheat the oven to 300 degrees F.
2. In a large Dutch oven, heat the oil over medium-high heat and stir fry the lamb necks with a little salt for about 4-5 minutes or until browned completely.
3. With a slotted spoon, transfer the lamb onto a plate and Now, reduce the heat to medium.
4. In the same pan, add the onion and sauté for about 10 minutes.
5. Add the ginger, garlic and spices and sauté for about 1 minute.
6. Add the yogurt and tomatoes and cook for about 3-4 minutes.
7. With an immersion blender, blend the mixture until smooth.
8. Add the lamb, boiling water and salt and bring to a boil.
9. Cover the pan and transfer into the oven.
10. Bake for about 2½ hours.
11. Now, remove the pan from oven and place over medium heat.
12. Stir in spinach and garam masala and cook for about 3-5 minutes.
13. Stir in lemon juice, salt and black pepper and remove from heat.
14. Serve hot.

Pork Salad

Cooking Time: 6 minutes
Serves: 5

Ingredients:
- 1½ pounds pork tenderloin, trimmed and sliced thinly
- Salt and ground black pepper, as required
- 3 tablespoon olive oil
- 2 carrots, peeled and grated
- 3 cups Napa cabbage, shredded
- 2 scallions, chopped
- 2 tablespoon fresh lime juice
- ¼ cup fresh mint leaves, chopped

Directions:
1. Season the pork with salt and black pepper lightly.
2. In a large skillet, heat the oil over medium heat and cook the pork slices for about 2-3 minutes per sides or until cooked through.
3. Remove from the heat and set aside to cool slightly.
4. In a large bowl, add the pork and remaining ingredients except mint leaves and toss to coat well. Serve with the garnishing of mint leaves.

Pork with Bell Peppers

Cooking Time: 13 minutes
Serves: 4

Ingredients:
- 1 tablespoon fresh ginger, chopped finely
- 4 garlic cloves, chopped finely
- 1 cup fresh cilantro, chopped and divided
- ¼ cup plus 1 tablespoon olive oil, divided
- 1 pound tender pork, trimmed, sliced thinly
- 2 onions, sliced thinly
- 1 green bell pepper, seeded and sliced thinly
- 1 red bell pepper, seeded and sliced thinly
- 1 tablespoon fresh lime juice

Directions:
1. In a large bowl, mix together ginger, garlic, ½ cup of cilantro and ¼ cup of oil.
2. Add the pork and coat with mixture generously.
3. Refrigerate to marinate for about 2 hours.
4. Heat a large skillet over medium-high heat and stir fry the pork mixture for about 4-5 minutes. Transfer the pork into a bowl.
5. In the same skillet, heat remaining oil over medium heat and sauté the onion for about 3 minutes. Stir in the bell pepper and stir fry for about 3 minutes.
6. Stir in the pork, lime juice and remaining cilantro and cook for about 2 minutes. Serve hot.

Roasted Pork Shoulder

Cooking Time: 6 hours

Serves: 12

Ingredients:

- 1 head garlic, peeled and crushed
- ¼ cup fresh rosemary, minced
- 2 tablespoons fresh lemon juice
- 2 tablespoons balsamic vinegar
- 1 (4-pound) pork shoulder, trimmed

Directions:

1. In a bowl, add all the ingredients except pork shoulder and mix well.
2. In a large roasting pan place pork shoulder and coat with marinade generously.
3. With a large plastic wrap, cover the roasting pan and refrigerate to marinate for at least 1-2 hours.
4. Remove the roasting pan from refrigerator.
5. Remove the plastic wrap from roasting pan and keep in room temperature for 1 hour.
6. Preheat the oven to 275 degrees F.
7. Arrange the roasting pan in oven and roast for about 6 hours.
8. Remove from the oven and set aside for about 15-20 minutes.
9. With a sharp knife, cut the pork shoulder into desired slices and serve.

Pork Chops in Peach Glaze

Cooking Time: 16 minutes

Serves: 2

Ingredients:

- 2 (6-ounce) boneless pork chops, trimmed
- Sea Salt and ground black pepper, as required
- ½ of ripe yellow peach, peeled, pitted and chopped
- 1 tablespoon olive oil
- 2 tablespoons shallot, minced
- 2 tablespoons garlic, minced
- 2 tablespoons fresh ginger, minced
- 4-6 drops liquid stevia
- 1 tablespoon balsamic vinegar
- ¼ teaspoon red pepper flakes, crushed
- ¼ cup filtered water

Directions:

1. Season the pork chops with sea salt and black pepper generously.
2. In a blender, add the peach pieces and pulse until a puree forms.
3. Reserve the remaining peach pieces.
4. In a skillet, heat the oil over medium heat and sauté the shallots for about 1-2 minutes.
5. Add the garlic and ginger and sauté for about 1 minute.
6. Stir in the remaining ingredients and bring to a boil.
7. Now, reduce the heat to medium-low and simmer for about 4-5 minutes or until a sticky glaze forms.
8. Remove from the heat and reserve 1/3 of the glaze and set aside.
9. Coat the chops with remaining glaze.
10. Heat a nonstick skillet over medium-high heat and sear the chops for about 4 minutes per side.
11. Transfer the chops onto a plate and coat with the remaining glaze evenly.
12. Serve immediately.

Ground Pork with Spinach

Cooking Time: 15 minutes

Serves: 4

Ingredients:

- 1 tablespoon olive oil
- ½ of white onion, chopped
- 2 garlic cloves, chopped finely
- 1 jalapeño pepper, chopped finely
- 1 pound lean ground pork
- 1 teaspoon ground coriander
- 1 teaspoon ground cumin
- ½ teaspoon ground turmeric
- ½ teaspoon ground cinnamon
- ½ teaspoon ground fennel seeds
- Salt and ground black pepper, as required
- ½ cup fresh cherry tomatoes, quartered
- 1¼ pounds collard greens leaves, stemmed and chopped
- 1 teaspoon fresh lemon juice

Directions:

1. In a large skillet, heat the oil over medium heat and sauté the onion for about 4 minutes.
2. Add the garlic and jalapeño pepper and sauté for about 1 minute.
3. Add the pork and spices and cook for about 6 minutes breaking into pieces with the spoon.
4. Stir in the tomatoes and greens and cook, stirring gently for about 4 minutes.
5. Stir in the lemon juice and remove from heat.
6. Serve hot.

Poultry Recipes

Chicken with Chickpeas

Cooking Time: 36 minutes

Serves: 4

Ingredients:

- 2 tablespoons olive oil
- 1 pound skinless, boneless chicken breast, cubed
- 2 carrots, peeled and sliced
- 1 onion, chopped
- 2 celery stalks, chopped
- 2 garlic cloves, chopped
- 1 tablespoon fresh ginger root, minced
- ½ teaspoon dried oregano, crushed
- ¾ teaspoon ground cumin
- ½ teaspoon paprika
- ¼-13 teaspoon cayenne pepper
- ¼ teaspoon ground turmeric
- 1 cup tomatoes, crushed
- 1½ cups low-sodium chicken broth
- 1 zucchini, sliced
- 1 cup boiled chickpeas, drained
- 1 tablespoon fresh lemon juice

Directions:
1. In a large nonstick pan, heat the oil over medium heat and cook the chicken cubes for about 4-5 minutes.
2. With a slotted spoon, transfer the chicken cubes onto a plate.
3. In the same pan, add the carrot, onion, celery and garlic and sauté for about 4-5 minutes.
4. Add the ginger, oregano and spices and sauté for about 1 minute.
5. Add the chicken, tomato and broth and bring to a boil.
6. Now, reduce the heat to low and simmer for about 10 minutes.
7. Add the zucchini and chickpeas and simmer, covered for about 15 minutes.
8. Stir in the lemon juice and serve hot.

Chicken & Broccoli Bake

Cooking Time: 45 minutes

Serves: 6

Ingredients:

- 6 (6-ounce) boneless, skinless chicken breasts
- 3 broccoli heads, cut into florets
- 4 garlic cloves, minced
- ¼ cup olive oil
- 1 teaspoon dried oregano, crushed
- 1 teaspoon dried rosemary, crushed
- Sea Salt and ground black pepper, as required

Directions:
1. Preheat the oven to 375 degrees F. Grease a large baking dish.
2. In a large bowl, add all the ingredients and toss to coat well.
3. In the bottom of prepared baking dish, arrange the broccoli florets and top with chicken breasts in a single layer.
4. Bake for about 45 minutes.
5. Remove from the oven and set aside for about 5 minutes before serving.

Meatballs Curry

Cooking Time: 25 minutes
Serves: 6

Ingredients:

For Meatballs:
- 1 pound lean ground chicken
- 1 tablespoon onion paste
- 1 teaspoons fresh ginger paste
- 1 teaspoons garlic paste
- 1 green chili, chopped finely
- 1 tablespoon fresh cilantro leaves, chopped
- 1 teaspoon ground coriander
- ½ teaspoon cumin seeds
- ½ teaspoon red chili powder
- ½ teaspoon ground turmeric
- 1/8 teaspoon salt

For Curry:
- 3 tablespoons olive oil
- ½ teaspoon cumin seeds
- 1 (1-inch) cinnamon stick
- 2 onions, chopped
- 1 teaspoons fresh ginger, minced
- 1 teaspoons garlic, minced
- 4 tomatoes, chopped finely
- 2 teaspoons ground coriander
- 1 teaspoon garam masala powder
- ½ teaspoon ground nutmeg
- ½ teaspoon red chili powder
- ½ teaspoon ground turmeric
- Salt, as required
- 1 cup filtered water
- 3 tablespoons fresh cilantro, chopped

Directions:
1. For meatballs: in a large bowl, add all ingredients and mix until well combined. Make small equal-sized meatballs from mixture.
2. In a large deep skillet, heat the oil over medium heat and cook the meatballs for about 3-5 minutes or until browned from all sides.
3. Transfer the meatballs into a bowl.
4. In the same skillet, add the cumin seeds and cinnamon stick and sauté for about 1 minute. Add the onions and sauté for about 4-5 minutes.
5. Add the ginger and garlic paste and sauté for about 1 minute.
6. Add the tomato and spices and cook, crushing with the back of spoon for about 2-3 minutes. Add the water and meatballs and bring to a boil.
7. Now, reduce the heat to low and simmer for about 10 minutes.
8. Serve hot with the garnishing of cilantro.

Chicken, Oats & Chickpeas Meatloaf

Cooking Time: 1¼ hours

Serves: 4

Ingredients:

- ½ cup cooked chickpeas
- 2 egg whites
- 2½ teaspoons poultry seasoning
- Ground black pepper, as required
- 10 ounce lean ground chicken
- 1 cup red bell pepper, seeded and minced
- 1 cup celery stalk, minced
- 1/3 cup steel-cut oats
- 1 cup tomato puree, divided
- 2 tablespoons dried onion flakes, crushed
- 1 tablespoon prepared mustard

Directions:
1. Preheat the oven to 350 degrees F. Grease a 9x5-inch loaf pan.
2. In a food processor, add chickpeas, egg whites, poultry seasoning and black pepper and pulse until smooth.
3. Transfer the mixture into a large bowl.
4. Add the chicken, veggies oats, ½ cup of tomato puree and onion flakes and mix until well combined.
5. Transfer the mixture into prepared loaf pan evenly.
6. With your hands, press, down the mixture slightly.
7. In another bowl mix together mustard and remaining tomato puree.
8. Place the mustard mixture over loaf pan evenly.
9. Bake for about 1-1¼ hours or until desired doneness.
10. Remove from the oven and set aside for about 5 minutes before slicing.g.
11. Cut into desired sized slices and serve.

Herbed Turkey Breast

Cooking Time: 1 hour 50 minutes

Serves: 6

Ingredients:

- ½ cup olive oil
- 2 tablespoons fresh lemon juice
- 1 tablespoon scallion, chopped
- ½ teaspoon dried marjoram, crushed
- ½ teaspoon dried sage, crushed
- ½ teaspoon dried thyme, crushed
- Salt and ground black pepper, as required
- 1 (2-pound) boneless, skinless turkey breast half

Directions:
1. Preheat the oven to 325 degrees F. Arrange a rack into a greased shallow roasting pan.
2. In a small pan, all the ingredients except turkey breast over medium heat and bring to a boil, stirring frequently.
3. Remove from the heat and set aside to cool.
4. Place turkey breast into the prepared roasting pan.
5. Place some of the herb mixture over the top of turkey breast.
6. Cover the roasting pan and bake for about 1¼-1¾ hours, basting with the remaining herb mixture occasionally.
7. Remove from the oven and set aside for about 10-15 minutes before slicing.
8. With a sharp knife, cut into desired slices and serve.

Turkey with Lentils

Cooking Time: 51 minutes

Serves: 7

Ingredients:

- 3 tablespoons olive oil, divided
- 1 onion, chopped
- 1 tablespoon fresh ginger, minced
- 4 garlic cloves, minced
- 3 plum tomatoes, chopped finely
- 2 cups dried red lentils, soaked for 30 minutes and drained
- 2 cups filtered water
- 2 teaspoons cumin seeds
- ½ teaspoon cayenne pepper
- 1 pound lean ground turkey
- 1 jalapeño pepper, seeded and chopped
- 2 scallions, chopped
- ¼ cup fresh cilantro, chopped

Directions:
1. In a Dutch oven, heat 1 tablespoon of oil over medium heat and sauté the onion, ginger and garlic for about 5 minutes.
2. Stir in tomatoes, lentils and water and bring to a boil
3. Now, reduce the heat to medium-low and simmer, covered for about 30 minutes.
4. Meanwhile, in a skillet, heat remaining oil over medium heat and sauté the cumin seeds and cayenne pepper for about 1 minute.
5. Transfer the mixture into a small bowl and set aside.
6. In the same skillet, add turkey and cook for about 4-5 minutes.
7. Add the jalapeño and scallion and cook for about 4-5 minutes.
8. Add the spiced oil mixture and stir to combine well.
9. Transfer the turkey mixture in simmering lentils and simmer for about 10-15 minutes or until desired doneness.
10. Serve hot.

Vegetarian Recipes

Baked Beans

Cooking Time: 2 hours 10 minutes

Serves: 4

Ingredients:

- ¼ pound dry lima beans, soaked overnight and drained
- ¼ pound dry red kidney beans, soaked overnight and drained
- 1¼ tablespoons 0ive oil
- 1 small onion, chopped
- 4 garlic cloves, minced
- 1 teaspoon dried thyme, crushed
- ½ teaspoon ground cumin
- ½ teaspoon red pepper flakes, crushed
- ¼ teaspoon paprika
- 1 tablespoon balsamic vinegar
- 1 cup homemade tomato puree
- 1 cup low-sodium vegetable broth
- Ground black pepper, as required
- 2 tablespoons fresh parsley, chopped

Directions:
1. In a large pan of the boiling water, add the beans over high heat and bring to a boil.
2. Now, reduce the heat to low and simmer, covered for about 1 hour.
3. Remove from the heat and drain the beans well.
4. Preheat the oven to 325 degrees F.
5. In a large ovenproof pan, heat the oil over medium heat and cook the onion for about 8-9 minutes, stirring frequently.
6. Add the garlic, thyme and red spices and sauté for about 1 minute.
7. Add the cooked beans and remaining ingredients and immediately remove from the heat.
8. Cover the pan and transfer into the oven.
9. Bake for about 1 hour.
10. Serve with the garnishing of cilantro.

Spicy Black Beans

Cooking Time: 1½ hours

Serves: 6

Ingredients:

- 4 cups filtered water
- 1½ cups dried black beans, soaked for 8 hours and drained
- ½ teaspoon ground turmeric
- 3 tablespoons olive oil
- 1 small onion, chopped finely
- 1 green chili, chopped
- 1 (1-inch) piece fresh ginger, minced
- 2 garlic cloves, minced
- 1-1½ tablespoons ground coriander
- 1 teaspoon ground cumin
- ½ teaspoon cayenne pepper
- Sea salt, as required
- 2 medium tomatoes, chopped finely
- ½ cup fresh cilantro, chopped

Directions:
1. In a large pan, add water, black beans and turmeric and bring to a boil on high heat.
2. Now, reduce the heat to low and simmer, covered for about 1 hour or till desired doneness of beans.
3. Meanwhile, in a skillet, heat the oil over medium heat and sauté the onion for about 4-5 minutes.
4. Add the green chili, ginger, garlic, spices and salt and sauté for about 1-2 minutes.
5. Stir in the tomatoes and cook for about 10 minutes, stirring occasionally.
6. Transfer the tomato mixture into the pan with black beans and stir to combine.
7. Increase the heat to medium-low and simmer for about 15-20 minutes.
8. Stir in the cilantro and simmer for about 5 minutes.
9. Serve hot.

Lentils Chili

Cooking Time: 2 hours 20 minutes

Serves: 8

Ingredients:

- 2 teaspoons olive oil
- 1 large onion, chopped
- 3 medium carrot, peeled and chopped
- 4 celery stalks, chopped
- 2 garlic cloves, minced
- 1 jalapeño pepper, seeded and chopped
- ½ tablespoon dried thyme, crushed
- 1 tablespoon chipotle chili powder
- ½ tablespoon cayenne pepper
- 1½ tablespoons ground coriander
- 1½ tablespoons ground cumin
- 1 teaspoon ground turmeric
- Ground black pepper, as required
- 1 tomato, chopped finely
- 1 pound lentils, rinsed
- 8 cups low-sodium vegetable broth
- 6 cups fresh spinach
- ½ cup fresh cilantro, chopped

Directions:
1. In a large pan, heat the oil over medium heat and sauté the onion, carrot and celery for about 5 minutes.
2. Add the garlic, jalapeño pepper, thyme and spices and sauté for about 1 minute.
3. Add the tomato paste, lentils and broth and bring to a boil.
4. Now, reduce the heat to low and simmer for about 2 hours.
5. Stir in the spinach and simmer for about 3-5 minutes.
6. Stir in cilantro and remove from the heat.
7. Serve hot.

Quinoa in Tomato Sauce

Cooking Time: 40 minutes
Serves: 4

Ingredients:
- 2 tablespoons olive oil
- 1 cup quinoa, rinsed
- 1 green bell pepper, seeded and chopped
- 1 medium onion, chopped finely
- 3 garlic cloves, minced
- 2½ cups filtered water
- 2 cups tomatoes, crushed finely
- 1 teaspoon red chili powder
- ¼ teaspoon ground cumin
- ¼ teaspoon garlic powder
- Ground black pepper, as required

Directions:
1. In a large pan, heat the oil over medium-high heat and cook the quinoa, onion, bell pepper and garlic for about 5 minutes, stirring frequently.
2. Stir in the remaining ingredients and bring to a boil.
3. Now, reduce the heat to medium-low.
4. Cover the pan tightly and simmer for about 3o minutes, stirring occasionally.
5. Serve hot.

Grains Combo

Cooking Time: 35 minutes
Serves: 6

Ingredients:
- ¾ cup amaranth
- 1 cup quinoa, rinsed
- ¼ cup wild rice
- 4¼ cups filtered water
- 2 teaspoons ground cumin
- ½ teaspoon paprika
- Salt, as required
- 1¼ cups boiled chickpeas
- 2 medium carrots, peeled and grated
- 1 garlic clove, minced
- Ground black pepper, as required

Directions:
1. In a large pan, add the amaranth, quinoa, wild rice, water and spices over medium-high heat and bring to a boil.
2. Now, reduce the heat to medium-low and simmer, covered for about 20-25 minutes. Stir in remaining ingredients and simmer for about 3-5 minutes.
3. Serve hot.

Barley Pilaf

Cooking Time: 1 hour 5 minutes

Serves: 4

Ingredients:

- ½ cup pearl barley
- 1 cup low-sodium vegetable broth
- 2 tablespoons olive oil, divided
- 2 garlic cloves, minced finely
- ½ cup onion, chopped
- ½ cup eggplant, sliced thinly
- ½ cup green bell pepper, seeded and chopped
- ½ cup red bell pepper, seeded and chopped
- 2 tablespoons fresh cilantro, chopped
- 2 tablespoons fresh mint leaves, chopped

Directions:

1. In a pan, add the barley and broth over medium-high heat and bring to a boil.
2. Immediately, reduce the heat to low and simmer, covered for about 45 minutes or until all the liquid is absorbed.
3. In a large skillet, heat 1 tablespoon of oil over high heat and sauté the garlic for about 1 minute.
4. Stir in the cooked barley and cook for about 3 minutes.
5. Remove from heat and set aside.
6. In another skillet, heat remaining oil over medium heat and sauté the onion for about 5-7 minutes.
7. Add the eggplant and bell peppers and stir fry for about 3 minutes.
8. Stir in the remaining ingredients except walnuts and cook for about 2-3 minutes.
9. Stir in barley mixture and cook for about 2-3 minutes.
10. Serve hot.

Baked Veggies Combo

Cooking Time: 40 minutes

Serves: 8

Ingredients:

- 2 large zucchinis, sliced
- 1 large yellow squash, sliced
- 3 cups fresh broccoli florets
- 1 pound fresh asparagus, trimmed
- 2 garlic cloves, minced
- 1 tablespoon fresh rosemary, minced
- 1 tablespoon fresh thyme, minced
- ½ teaspoon ground cumin
- ½ teaspoon red pepper flakes, crushed
- ¼ teaspoon cayenne pepper
- 2 tablespoons olive oil
- Salt, as required

Directions:

1. Preheat the oven to 400 degrees F. Line 2 large baking sheets with aluminum foil.
2. In a large bowl, add all ingredients and toss to coat well.
3. Divide the vegetables mixture onto prepared baking sheets and spread in a single layer.
4. Roast for about 35-40 minutes.
5. Remove from oven and serve.

Mixed Veggie Salad

Cooking Time: 20 minutes

Serves: 8

Ingredients:

For Dressing:

- 1/3 cup olive oil
- ½ cup fresh lemon juice
- 1 tablespoon fresh ginger, grated
- 2 teaspoons mustard
- 4-6 drops liquid stevia
- ¼ teaspoon salt

For Salad:

- 2 avocados, peeled, pitted and chopped
- 2 tablespoons fresh lemon juice
- 2 cups fresh baby spinach, torn
- 2 cups small broccoli florets
- 1 cup red cabbage, shredded
- 1 cup purple cabbage, shredded
- 2 large carrots, peeled and grated
- 1 small orange bell pepper, seeded and sliced into matchsticks
- 1 small yellow bell pepper, seeded and sliced into matchsticks
- ½ cup fresh parsley leaves, chopped
- 1 cup walnuts, chopped

Directions:

1. For dressing: in a food processor, add all ingredients and pulse until well combined.
2. In a large bowl, add the avocado slices and drizzle with lemon juice.
3. Add the remaining vegetables and mix.
4. Place the dressing and toss to coat well.
5. Serve immediately.

Tofu with Brussels Sprout

Cooking Time: 15 minutes

Serves: 4

Ingredients:

- 1 tablespoon olive oil, divided
- 8 ounces extra-firm tofu, drained, pressed and cut into slices
- 2 garlic cloves, chopped
- 1/3 cup pecans, toasted and chopped
- 1 tablespoon unsweetened applesauce
- ¼ cup fresh cilantro, chopped
- ¾ pound Brussels sprouts, trimmed and cut into wide ribbons

Directions:

1. In a skillet, heat ½ tablespoon of the oil over medium heat and sauté the tofu and for about 6-7 minutes or until golden brown.
2. Add the garlic and pecans and sauté for about 1 minute.
3. Add the applesauce and cook for about 2 minutes.
4. Stir in the cilantro and remove from heat.
5. Transfer tofu into a plate and set aside
6. In the same skillet, heat the remaining oil over medium-high heat and cook the Brussels sprouts for about 5 minutes.
7. Stir in the tofu and remove from the heat.
8. Serve immediately.

Beans, Walnuts & Veggie Burgers

Cooking Time: 25 minutes

Serves: 8

Ingredients:

- ½ cup walnuts
- 1 carrot, peeled and chopped
- 1 celery stalk, chopped
- 4 scallions, chopped
- 5 garlic cloves, chopped
- 2¼ cups cooked black beans
- 2½ cups sweet potato, peeled and grated
- ½ teaspoon red pepper flakes, crushed
- ¼ teaspoon cayenne pepper
- Salt and ground black pepper, as required

Directions:

1. Preheat the oven to 400 degrees F. Line a baking sheet with parchment paper.
2. In a food processor, add walnuts and pulse until finely ground.
3. Add the carrot, celery, scallion and garlic and pulse until chopped finely.
4. Transfer the vegetable mixture into a large bowl.
5. In the same food processor, add beans and pulse until chopped.
6. Add 1½ cups of sweet potato and pulse until a chunky mixture forms.
7. Transfer the bean mixture into the bowl with vegetable mixture.
8. Stir in the remaining sweet potato and spices and mix until well combined.
9. Make 8 patties from mixture.
10. Arrange the patties onto prepared baking sheet in a single layer.
11. Bake for about 25 minutes.
12. Serve hot.

Side Recipes

Spicy Spinach

Cooking Time: 20 minutes   Serves: 3

Ingredients:
- 1 tablespoon olive oil
- 1 red onion, chopped finely
- 6 garlic cloves, minced
- 1 (1-inch) piece fresh ginger, minced
- 1 teaspoon garam masala
- 1 teaspoon ground coriander
- ½ teaspoon ground cumin
- ¼ teaspoon ground turmeric
- 6 cups fresh spinach, chopped
- Salt and ground black pepper, as required
- 1-2 tablespoons water

Directions:
1. Heat the olive oil in a large nonstick skillet over medium heat and sauté the onion for about 6-7 minutes.
2. Add the garlic, ginger and spices and sauté for about 1 minute.
3. Add the spinach, salt and black pepper and water and cook, covered for about 10 minutes.
4. Uncover and stir fry for about 2 minutes. 5.Serve hot.

Herbed Asparagus

Cooking Time: 10 minutes   Serves: 4

Ingredients:
- 2 tablespoons olive oil
- 2 tablespoons fresh lemon juice
- 1 tablespoon balsamic vinegar
- 1 teaspoon garlic, minced
- 1 tablespoon fresh parsley, chopped
- 1 teaspoon dried oregano
- Salt and ground black pepper, as required
- 1 pound fresh asparagus, ends removed

Directions:
1. Preheat oven to 400 degrees F and lightly grease a rimmed baking sheet.
2. Place the oil, lemon juice, vinegar, garlic, herbs, salt and black pepper in a bowl and beat until well combined.
3. Arrange the asparagus onto the prepared baking sheet in a single layer.
4. Top with half of the herb mixture and toss to coat.
5. Roast for about 8-10 minutes.
6. Remove from the oven and transfer the asparagus onto a platter.
7. Drizzle with the remaining herb mixture and serve.

Lemony Brussels Sprout

Cooking Time: 7 minutes Serves: 2

Ingredients:
- ½ pound Brussels sprouts, halved
- 1 tablespoon olive oil
- 1 garlic clove, minced
- ½ teaspoon red pepper flakes, crushed
- Salt and ground black pepper, as required
- 1 tablespoon fresh lemon juice

Directions:
1. Heat the olive oil in a large skillet over medium heat and cook the garlic and red pepper flakes for about 1 minute, stirring continuously.
2. Stir in the Brussels sprouts, salt and black pepper and sauté for about 4-5 minutes.
3. Stir in lemon juice and sauté for about 1 minute more.
4. Serve hot.

Gingered Cauliflower

Cooking Time: 0 minutes Serves: 2

Ingredients:
- 2 cups cauliflower, cut into 1-inch florets
- Salt, as required
- 2 tablespoons olive oil
- 1 teaspoon fresh ginger root, sliced thinly
- 2 fresh thyme sprigs

Directions:
1. In a pan of the water, add the cauliflower and salt over medium heat and bring to a boil.
2. Cover and cook for about 10-12 minutes.
3. Drain the cauliflower well and transfer onto a serving platter.
4. Meanwhile, in a small skillet, melt the coconut oil over medium-low heat.
5. Add the ginger and thyme sprigs and swirl the pan occasionally for about 2-3 minutes.
6. Discard the ginger and thyme sprigs.
7. Pour the oil over cauliflower and serve immediately.

Roasted Broccoli

Cooking Time: 15 minutes   Serves: 2

Ingredients:
- 2 cups fresh broccoli florets
- 1 small yellow onion, cut into wedges
- ¼ teaspoon garlic powder
- 1/8 teaspoon paprika
- 1/8 teaspoon freshly ground black pepper
- 2 tablespoons olive oil

Directions:
1. Preheat the grill to medium heat.
2. In a large bowl, add all the ingredients and toss to coat well.
3. Transfer the broccoli mixture over a double thickness of a foil paper.
4. Fold the foil paper around broccoli mixture to seal it.
5. Grill for about 10-15 minutes.
6. Serve hot.

Garlicky Cabbage

Cooking Time: 10 minutes
Serves: 4

Ingredients:
- 1 tablespoon olive oil
- 2 garlic cloves, minced
- 1 pound cabbage, shredded
- 2-3 tablespoons filtered water
- 1½ tablespoons fresh lemon juice
- Salt and ground black pepper, as required

Directions:
1. In a large skillet, heat the oil over medium heat and sauté the garlic for about 1 minute.
2. Stir in the cabbage and cook, covered for about 2-3 minute.
3. Stir in the water and cook for about 2-3 minutes, stirring continuously.
4. Increase the heat to high and stir in the lemon juice, salt and black pepper.
5. Cook for about 2-3 minutes, stirring continuously. Serve hot.

Stir Fried Zucchini

Cooking Time: 10 minutes
Serves: 4

Ingredients:
- 1 tablespoon olive oil
- ½ cup yellow onion, sliced
- 4 cups zucchini, sliced
- 1½ teaspoons garlic, minced
- ¼ cup water
- Salt and ground black pepper, as required

Directions:
1. In a large skillet, heat the oil over medium-high heat and sauté the onion and zucchini for about 4-5 minutes.
2. Add the garlic and sauté for about 1 minute.
3. Add the remaining ingredients and stir to combine.
4. Now, reduce the heat to medium and cook for about 3-4 minutes, stirring occasionally.
5. Serve hot.

Green Beans with Tomatoes

Cooking Time: 40 minutes
Serves: 8

Ingredients:
- ¼ teaspoon fresh lemon peel, grated finely
- 2 teaspoons olive oil
- Salt and freshly ground white pepper, as required
- 4 cups grape tomatoes
- 1½ pounds fresh green beans, trimmed

Directions:
1. Preheat the oven to 350 degrees F.
2. In a large bowl, mix together lemon peel, oil, salt and white pepper.
3. Add the cherry tomatoes and toss to coat well.
4. Transfer the tomato mixture into a roasting pan.
5. Roast for about 35-40 minutes, stirring once in the middle way.
6. Meanwhile, in a pan of boiling water, arrange a steamer basket.
7. Place the green beans in steamer basket and steam, covered for about 7-8 minutes.
8. Drain the green beans well.
9. Divide the green beans and tomatoes onto serving plates and serve.

French Green Beans

Cooking Time: 5 minutes
Serves: 4

Ingredients:
- Water
- 2 cups green beans, rinsed, drained and trimmed
- 1 tablespoon shallot, minced
- 2 teaspoons olive oil
- 2 teaspoons fresh thyme, chopped
- Salt and pepper to taste

Directions:
1. Put a steamer basket in a large pan.
2. Add water to the bottom of the pan.
3. Bring it to a boil.
4. Put the beans on top of the basket and cover.
5. Reduce heat and steam for 2 minutes.
6. Drain and then rinse with cold water.
7. In a bowl, mix the rest of the ingredients.
8. Toss the beans in the mixture.

Roasted Summer Squash

Cooking Time: 15 minutes
Serves: 4

Ingredients:
- Cooking spray
- 2 summer squash, sliced into strips
- 1 ½ teaspoons olive oil
- Garlic salt and pepper to taste
- Parmesan cheese

Directions:
1. Preheat your oven to 425 degrees F.
2. Line a baking sheet with foil
3. Spray oil on the foil.
4. Toss the squash strips in the olive oil and season with salt and pepper.
5. Arrange on a single layer on the pan.
6. Roast for 15 minutes.
7. Sprinkle with Parmesan cheese before serving.

Veggie Mash

Cooking Time: 35 minutes
Serves: 4

Ingredients:
- 1 onion, sliced into wedges
- 2 cloves garlic, sliced in half
- 2 carrots, sliced into wedges
- 1 sweet potato, sliced into strips
- 4 teaspoons olive oil
- Salt and pepper to taste
- 1 teaspoon fresh ginger, grated
- 3 tablespoons nonfat milk

Directions:
1. Preheat your oven to 425 degrees F.
2. Put the onion, garlic, carrots and sweet potato in a baking pan.
3. Drizzle with oil and toss to coat evenly.
4. Cover with foil and roast for 25 minutes.
5. Take the vegetables out of the foil and roast for another 10 minutes.
6. Transfer to a food processor.
7. Add the salt, pepper and ginger.
8. Pulse until smooth.
9. Gradually add milk until desired consistency is achieved.

Mushroom Medley

Cooking Time: 25 minutes
Serves: 6

Ingredients:
- 1 lb. assorted fresh mushrooms, sliced
- 6 cloves garlic, sliced thinly
- 2 teaspoons balsamic vinegar
- 2 tablespoons olive oil
- 2 tablespoons fresh Italian parsley, chopped
- 2 teaspoons Worcestershire sauce
- 1 teaspoon dried oregano, crushed
- Salt and pepper to taste

Directions:
1. Preheat your oven to 400 degrees F.
2. Put the mushrooms on a baking sheet. Stir in the garlic slices.
3. In a bowl, mix the vinegar, olive oil and Worcestershire sauce.
4. Toss the mushroom and garlic in this mixture.
5. Season with oregano, salt and pepper.
6. Roast for 25 minutes.
7. Sprinkle parsley on top before serving.

Fish And Seafood Recipes

Salmon Soup

Cooking Time: 20 minutes
Serves: 4

Ingredients:
- 1 tablespoon olive oil
- 1 yellow onion, chopped
- 1 garlic clove, minced
- 4 cups low-sodium chicken broth
- 1 pound boneless salmon, cubed
- 2 tablespoon fresh cilantro, chopped
- Ground black pepper, as required
- 1 tablespoon fresh lime juice

Directions:
1. In a large pan heat the oil over medium heat and sauté the onion for about 5 minutes.
2. Add the garlic and sauté for about 1 minute.
3. Stir in the broth and bring to a boil over high heat.
4. Now, reduce the heat to low and simmer for about 10 minutes.
5. Add the salmon, and soy sauce and cook for about 3-4 minutes.
6. Stir in black pepper, lime juice, and cilantro and serve hot.

Salmon & Shrimp Stew

Cooking Time: 21 minutes
Serves: 6

Ingredients:
- 2 tablespoons olive oil
- ½ cup onion, chopped finely
- 2 garlic cloves, minced
- 1 Serrano pepper, chopped
- 1 teaspoon smoked paprika
- 4 cups fresh tomatoes, chopped
- 4 cups low-sodium chicken broth
- 1 pound salmon fillets, cubed
- 1 pound shrimp, peeled and deveined
- 2 tablespoons fresh lime juice
- ¼ cup fresh basil, chopped
- ¼ cup fresh parsley, chopped
- Ground black pepper, as required
- 2 scallions, chopped

Directions:
1. In a large soup pan, melt coconut oil over medium-high heat and sauté the onion for about 5-6 minutes.
2. Add the garlic, Serrano pepper and smoked paprika and sauté for about 1 minute.
3. Add the tomatoes and broth and bring to a gentle simmer over medium heat.
4. Simmer for about 5 minutes.
5. Add the salmon and simmer for about 3-4 minutes.
6. Stir in the remaining seafood and cook for about 4-5 minutes.
7. Stir in the lemon juice, basil, parsley, sea salt and black pepper and remove from heat.
8. Serve hot with the garnishing of scallion.

Salmon Curry

Cooking Time: 30 minutes
Serves: 6

Ingredients:

- 6 (4-ounce) salmon fillets
- 1 teaspoon ground turmeric, divided
- Salt, as required
- 3 tablespoon olive oil, divided
- 1 yellow onion, chopped finely
- 1 teaspoon garlic paste
- 1 teaspoon fresh ginger paste
- 3-4 green chilies, halved
- 1 teaspoon red chili powder
- ½ teaspoon ground cumin
- ½ teaspoon ground cinnamon
- ¾ cup fat-free plain Greek yogurt, whipped
- ¾ cup filtered water
- 3 tablespoon fresh cilantro, chopped

Directions:

1. Season each salmon fillet with ½ teaspoon of the turmeric and salt.
2. In a large skillet, melt 1 tablespoon of the butter over medium heat and cook the salmon fillets for about 2 minutes per side.
3. Transfer the salmon onto a plate.
4. In the same skillet, melt the remaining butter over medium heat and sauté the onion for about 4-5 minutes.
5. Add the garlic paste, ginger paste, green chilies, remaining turmeric and spices and sauté for about 1 minute.
6. Now, reduce the heat to medium-low.
7. Slowly, add the yogurt and water, stirring continuously until smooth.
8. Cover the skillet and simmer for about 10-15 minutes or until desired doneness of the sauce.
9. Carefully, add the salmon fillets and simmer for about 5 minutes.
10. Serve hot with the garnishing of cilantro.

Salmon with Bell Peppers

Cooking Time: 20 minutes
Serves: 6

Ingredients:
- 6 (3-ounce) salmon fillets
- Pinch of salt
- Ground black pepper, as required
- 1 yellow bell pepper, seeded and cubed
- 1 red bell pepper, seeded and cubed
- 4 plum tomatoes, cubed
- 1 small onion, sliced thinly
- ½ cup fresh parsley, chopped
- ¼ cup olive oil
- 2 tablespoons fresh lemon juice

Directions:
1. Preheat the oven to 400 degrees F.
2. Season each salmon fillet with salt and black pepper lightly.
3. In a bowl, mix together the bell peppers, tomato and onion.
4. Arrange 6 foil pieces onto a smooth surface.
5. Place 1 salmon fillet over each foil paper and sprinkle with salt and black pepper.
6. Place veggie mixture over each fillet evenly and top with parsley and capers evenly.
7. Drizzle with oil and lemon juice.
8. Fold each foil around salmon mixture to seal it.
9. Arrange the foil packets onto a large baking sheet in a single layer.
10. Bake for about 20 minutes.
11. Serve hot.

Shrimp Salad

Cooking Time: 4 minutes
Serves: 6

Ingredients:

For Salad:
- 1 pound shrimp, peeled and deveined
- Salt and ground black pepper, as required
- 1 teaspoon olive oil
- 1½ cups carrots, peeled and julienned
- 1½ cups red cabbage, shredded
- 1½ cup cucumber, julienned
- 5 cups fresh baby arugula
- ¼ cup fresh basil, chopped
- ¼ cup fresh cilantro, chopped
- 4 cups lettuce, torn
- ¼ cup almonds, chopped

For Dressing:
- 2 tablespoons natural almond butter
- 1 garlic clove, crushed
- 1 tablespoon fresh cilantro, chopped
- 1 tablespoon fresh lime juice
- 1 tablespoon unsweetened applesauce
- 2 teaspoons balsamic vinegar
- ½ teaspoon cayenne pepper
- Salt, as required
- 1 tablespoon water
- 1/3 cup olive oil

Directions:
1. Slowly, add the oil, beating continuously until smooth.
2. For salad: in a bowl, add shrimp, salt, black pepper and oil and toss to coat well.
3. Heat a skillet over medium-high heat and cook the shrimp for about 2 minutes per side.
4. Remove from the heat and set aside to cool.
5. In a large bowl, add the shrimp, vegetables and mix well.
6. For dressing: in a bowl, add all ingredients except oil and beat until well combined.
7. Place the dressing over shrimp mixture and gently, toss to coat well.
8. Serve immediately.

Shrimp & Veggies Curry

Cooking Time: 20 minutes
Serves: 6

Ingredients:
- 2 teaspoons olive oil
- 1½ medium white onions, sliced
- 2 medium green bell peppers, seeded and sliced
- 3 medium carrots, peeled and sliced thinly
- 3 garlic cloves, chopped finely
- 1 tablespoon fresh ginger, chopped finely
- 2½ teaspoons curry powder
- 1½ pounds shrimp, peeled and deveined
- 1 cup filtered water
- 2 tablespoons fresh lime juice
- Salt and ground black pepper, as required
- 2 tablespoons fresh cilantro, chopped

Directions:
1. In a large skillet, heat oil over medium-high heat and sauté the onion for about 4-5 minutes.
2. Add the bell peppers and carrot and sauté for about 3-4 minutes.
3. Add the garlic, ginger and curry powder and sauté for about 1 minute.
4. Add the shrimp and sauté for about 1 minute.
5. Stir in the water and cook for about 4-6 minutes, stirring occasionally.
6. Stir in lime juice and remove from heat.
7. Serve hot with the garnishing of cilantro.

Shrimp with Zucchini

Cooking Time: 8 minutes
Serves: 4
Ingredients:
- 3 tablespoons olive oil
- 1 pound medium shrimp, peeled and deveined
- 1 shallot, minced
- 4 garlic cloves, minced
- ¼ teaspoon red pepper flakes, crushed
- Salt and ground black pepper, as required
- ¼ cup low-sodium chicken broth
- 2 tablespoons fresh lemon juice
- 1 teaspoon fresh lemon zest, grated finely
- ½ pound zucchini, spiralized with Blade C

Directions:
1. In a large skillet, heat the oil and butter over medium-high heat and cook the shrimp, shallot, garlic, red pepper flakes, salt and black pepper for about 2 minutes, stirring occasionally.
2. Stir in the broth, lemon juice and lemon zest and bring to a gentle boil.
3. Stir in zucchini noodles and cook for about 1-2 minutes.
4. Serve hot.

Shrimp with Broccoli

Cooking Time: 12 minutes   Serves: 6
Ingredients:
- 2 tablespoons olive oil, divided
- 4 cups broccoli, chopped
- 2-3 tablespoons filtered water
- 1½ pounds large shrimp, peeled and deveined
- 2 garlic cloves, minced
- 1 (1-inch) piece fresh ginger, minced
- Salt and ground black pepper, as required

Directions:
1. In a large skillet, heat 1 tablespoon of oil over medium-high heat and cook the broccoli for about 1-2 minutes stirring continuously.
2. Stir in the water and cook, covered for about 3-4 minutes, stirring occasionally.
3. With a spoon, push the broccoli to side of the pan.
4. Add the remaining oil and let it heat.
5. Add the shrimp and cook for about 1-2 minutes, tossing occasionally.
6. Add the remaining ingredients and sauté for about 2-3 minutes.
7. Serve hot.

Grilled Salmon with Ginger Sauce

Cooking Time: 8 minutes
Serves: 4

Ingredients:
- 1 tablespoon toasted sesame oil
- 1 tablespoon fresh cilantro, chopped
- 1 tablespoon lime juice
- 1 teaspoon fish sauce
- 1 clove garlic, mashed
- 1 teaspoon fresh ginger, grated
- 1 teaspoon jalapeño pepper, minced
- 4 salmon fillets
- 1 tablespoon olive oil
- Salt and pepper to taste

Directions:
1. In a bowl, mix the sesame oil, cilantro, lime juice, fish sauce, garlic, ginger and jalapeño pepper.
2. Preheat your grill.
3. Brush oil on salmon.
4. Season both sides with salt and pepper.
5. Grill salmon for 6 to 8 minutes, turning once or twice.
6. Take 1 tablespoon from the oil mixture.
7. Brush this on the salmon while grilling.
8. Serve grilled salmon with the remaining sauce.

Dessert Recipes

SUGAR FREE BUCKEYE BALLS

Cooking Time: 35 minutes
Serves: 36 balls

Ingredients:
- 6 cups of Sugar Free Powdered Sugar
- 1 teaspoon of Vanilla Extract
- 1 1/2 cups of Sugar Free Peanut Butter
- 1 cup of Butter very soft
- 4 cups of Sugar Free Chocolate Chips

Directions:
1. Prepare a baking sheet with wax paper. Set it aside.
2. Cream together the sugar-free peanut butter, vanilla extract and sugar free powdered sugar in a mixing bowl.
3. Form the mixture into 1 - 1 1/2-inches balls by rolling the dough in your hands.
4. Place each of the ball on the wax prepared baking sheet.
5. Place the prepared balls into the freezer for about 25 minutes, until hard.
6. Melt the chocolate in a microwave when you're ready to dip the balls in the chocolate or using the double boiler method.
7. Stir well as the chocolate melts.
8. Remove the peanut butter balls from the freezer and dip each of it into the chocolate. You can leave the area around where you put your toothpick.
9. Then place each ball back onto the wax paper and refrigerate them.
10. Melt more if you run low on chocolate.
11. Serve and enjoy.

PEANUT BUTTER COOKIES

Cooking Time: 15 mins
Serves: 12 balls

Ingredients:
- 1/2 teaspoon of baking soda
- 1/2 teaspoon of vanilla essence
- 1 cup of smooth peanut butter (no added sugar)
- 1 large egg
- 2/3 cup of erythritol

Directions:
1. Preheat oven to 350 degrees F.
2. Line a cookie tray with baking paper and set it aside.
3. Add the erythritol to a blender and blend until powdered. Set it aside. (Skip this step if using a confectioner's low carb sweetener).
4. In a medium mixing bowl, add all of the ingredients and mix until smooth and glossy dough forms.
5. Roll about 2 tablespoons of dough in your palms to form a ball, and place on the prepared cookie tray. Repeat until you consume the doughs. You will end up with 12 to 14 cookies.
6. Use a fork to flatten the cookies and create a criss cross patten across the top.
7. Bake the cookies for about 12 minutes.
8. Remove from the oven and allow it to cool on the baking tray, for about 25 minutes.
9. Transfer into a cooling rack for another 15 minutes.
10. Serve and enjoy.

CHOCOLATE FUDGE

Cooking Time: 2 hours
Serves: 40 squares

Ingredients:
- 10 ounces of bittersweet chocolate chips
- Optional: coarse or flaked sea salt for topping
- 1 1/2 cups of coconut butter
- 1 (13.66 FL ounces) can of full-fat coconut milk

Directions:
1. Use paper or foil to line an 8 by 8 inch baking pan.
2. Melt the coconut butter in a small saucepan over low heat.
3. Stir in the chocolate chips and coconut milk.
4. Cook over low heat, stirring consistently, until the chocolate chips are melted.
5. Pour the mixture into the pan.
6. Place in refrigerator for about 2 hours, until set.
7. Slice, serve and enjoy.

LOW-CARB CHEESECAKE

Cooking Time: 50 mins   Serves: 2 servings

Ingredients:
- 1 tablespoon of Stevia
- 1 teaspoon of vanilla extract
- 8.5 ounces of low fat cottage cheese
- 2 egg whites
- 1 scoop of vanilla protein powder
- 1 serving sugar-free Strawberry Jell-O
- Water

Directions:
1. Preheat the oven to 325 degrees F.
2. Prepare the Jell-O according to the instructions on the package.
3. Place in the freezer.
4. Blend egg whites and cottage cheese until the consistency is smooth.
5. Pour the blended mixture inside the bowl.
6. Whisk it together with the stevia, protein powder and vanilla extract.
7. Transfer the batter into a small nonstick pan, then bake for about 25 minutes.
8. Turn off the oven (but let the cake in it cool down).
9. Remove the cheesecake once the oven has cooled.
10. Pour it over the cheesecake when the Jell-O is almost set.
11. Let the cake set in the fridge for about 10 hours before enjoying.
12. Now you can serve and enjoy.

Chocolate & Raspberry Ice Cream

Cooking Time: 0 minutes
Serves: 8
Ingredients:
- ¼ cup almond milk
- 2 egg yolks
- 2 tablespoons cornstarch
- ¼ cup honey
- ¼ teaspoon almond extract
- ⅛ teaspoon salt
- 1 cup fresh raspberries
- 2 oz. dark chocolate, chopped
- ¼ cup almonds, slivered and toasted

Directions:
1. Mix almond milk, egg yolks, cornstarch and honey in a bowl.
2. Pour into a saucepan over medium heat.
3. Cook for 8 minutes.
4. Strain through a sieve.
5. Stir in salt and almond extract.
6. Chill for 8 hours.
7. Put into an ice cream maker.
8. Follow manufacturer's directions.
9. Stir in the rest of the ingredients.
10. Freeze for 4 hours.

Mocha Pops

Cooking Time: 0 minutes
Serves: 15
Ingredients:
- 3 cups brewed coffee
- ½ cup low calorie chocolate flavored syrup
- ¾ cup low fat half and half

Directions:
1. Mix the ingredients in a bowl.
2. Pour into popsicle molds.
3. Freeze for 4 hours.

Choco Banana Bites

Cooking Time: 5 minutes
Serves: 4
Ingredients:
- 2 bananas, sliced into rounds
- ¼ cup dark chocolate cubes

Directions:
1. Melt chocolate in the microwave or in a saucepan over medium heat.
2. Coat each banana slice with melted chocolate.
3. Place on a metal pan.
4. Freeze for 2 hours.

Blueberries with Yogurt

Cooking Time: 0 minute
Serves: 1
Ingredients:
- 1 cup nonfat Greek yogurt
- ¼ cup blueberries
- ¼ cup almonds

Directions:
1. Add yogurt and blueberries in a food processor.
2. Pulse until smooth.
3. Top with almonds before serving.

Fruit Kebab

Cooking Time: 0 minutes
Serves: 12
Ingredients:
- 3 apples
- ¼ cup orange juice
- 1 ½ lb. watermelon
- ¾ cup blueberries

Directions:
1. Use a star-shaped cookie cutter to cut out stars from the apple and watermelon.
2. Soak the apple stars in orange juice.
3. Thread the apple stars, watermelon stars and blueberries into skewers.
4. Refrigerate for 30 minutes before serving.

Roasted Mangoes

Cooking Time: 10 minutes
Serves: 4
Ingredients:
- 2 mangoes, peeled and sliced into cubes
- 2 tablespoons coconut flakes
- 2 teaspoons crystallized ginger, chopped
- 2 teaspoons orange zest

Directions:
1. Preheat your oven to 350 degrees F.
2. Put the mango cubes in custard cups.
3. Top with the ginger and orange zest.
4. Bake in the oven for 10 minutes.

Figs with Yogurt

Cooking Time: 0 minutes
Serves: 2

Ingredients:
- 8 oz. low fat yogurt
- ½ teaspoon vanilla
- 2 figs, sliced
- 1 tablespoon walnuts, toasted and chopped
- Lemon zest

Directions:
1. Refrigerate yogurt in a bowl for 8 hours.
2. After 8 hours, take it out of the refrigerator and stir in yogurt and vanilla.
3. Stir in the figs.
4. Sprinkle walnuts and lemon zest on top before serving.

Grilled Peaches

Cooking Time: 3 minutes
Serves: 6

Ingredients:
- 1 cup balsamic vinegar
- ⅛ teaspoon ground cinnamon
- 1 tablespoon honey
- 3 peaches, pitted and sliced in half
- 2 teaspoons olive oil
- 6 gingersnaps, crushed

Directions:
1. Pour the vinegar into a saucepan.
2. Bring it to a boil.
3. Lower heat and simmer for 10 minutes.
4. Remove from the stove.
5. Stir in cinnamon and honey.
6. Coat the peaches with oil.
7. Grill peaches for 2 to 3 minutes.
8. Drizzle each one with syrup.
9. Top with the gingersnaps.

Fruit Salad

Cooking Time: 0 minute
Serves: 6

Ingredients:
- 8 oz. light cream cheese
- 6 oz. Greek yogurt
- 1 tablespoon honey
- 1 teaspoon orange zest
- 1 teaspoon lemon zest
- 1 orange, sliced into sections
- 3 kiwi fruit, peeled and sliced
- 1 mango, cubed
- 1 cup blueberries

Directions:
1. Beat cream cheese using an electric mixer.
2. Add yogurt and honey.
3. Beat until smooth.
4. Stir in the orange and lemon zest.
5. Toss the fruits to mix.
6. Divide in glass jars.
7. Top with the cream cheese mixture.

30 - day meal plan

Day 1

Breakfast

Bell Pepper Pancakes

Lunch

Tortilla Chicken Soup

Dinner

French Lentils

Day 2

Breakfast

Sweet Potato Waffles

Lunch

Lamb Stew

Dinner

Chicken Fajitas

Day 3

Breakfast

Quinoa Bread

Lunch

Black Bean Salad

Dinner

Veggie Rice

Day 4

Breakfast

Tofu Scramble

Lunch

Kale Salad With Lemon Dressing

Dinner

Grilled Tuna Kebabs

Day 5

Breakfast

Apple Omelet

Lunch

Carrot Ginger Soup

Dinner

Spicy Turkey Tacos

Day 6

Breakfast

Veggie Frittata

Lunch

Shrimp Salad

Dinner

Lime Quinoa With Cilantro

Day 7

Breakfast

Chicken & Sweet Potato Hash

Lunch

Crispy Tofu

Dinner

Potatoes With Roasted Veggies

Day 8

Breakfast

Mini Veggie Quiche

Lunch

Spinach Soup With Pesto & Chicken

Dinner

Mushroom Stroganoff

Day 9

Breakfast

Shakshuka

Lunch

Asian Cold Noodle Salad

Dinner

Almond-Crusted Salmon

Day 10

Breakfast

Healthy Granola

Lunch

Beef Salad

Dinner

Chicken with Chickpeas

Day 11

Breakfast

Cinnamon Oatmeal Muffins With Apple

Lunch

Beef Curry

Dinner

Chicken & Broccoli Bake

Day 12

Breakfast

Veggie Omelet

Lunch

Beef with Barley & Veggies

Dinner

Meatballs Curry

Day 13

Breakfast

Spinach Scramble

Lunch

Beef with Broccoli

Dinner

Chicken, Oats & Chickpeas Meatloaf

Day 14

Breakfast

Breakfast Parfait

Lunch

Herbed Turkey Breast

Dinner

Ground Pork with Spinach

Day 15

Breakfast

Asparagus & Cheese Omelet

Lunch

Pork Chops in Peach Glaze

Dinner

Spicy Spinach

Day 16

Breakfast

Baked Beans

Lunch

Turkey with Lentils

Dinner

Roasted Pork Shoulder

Day 17

Breakfast

Grains Combo

Lunch

Pork with Bell Peppers

Dinner

Lamb Stew

Day 18

Breakfast

Sugar Free Buckeye Balls

Lunch

Herbed Asparagus

Dinner

Salmon Soup

Day 19

Breakfast

Peanut Butter Cookies

Lunch

Salmon & Shrimp Stew

Dinner

Mushroom Medley

Day 20

Breakfast

Low-Carb Cheesecake

Lunch

Gingered Cauliflower

Dinner

Pork Salad

Day 21

Breakfast

Baked Veggies Combo

Lunch

Salmon Curry

Dinner

Beans, Walnuts & Veggie Burgers

Day 22

Breakfast

Roasted Summer Squash

Lunch

Lemony Brussels Sprout

Dinner

Baked Lamb & Spinach

Day 23

Breakfast

Blueberries With Yogurt

Lunch

Salmon With Bell Peppers

Dinner

Fruit Salad

Day 24

Breakfast

Garlicky Cabbage

Lunch

Shrimp Salad

Dinner

French Green Beans

Day 25

Breakfast

Mixed Veggie Salad

Lunch

Spiced Leg Of Lamb

Dinner

Pan Grilled Steak

Day 26

Breakfast

Tofu With Brussels Sprout

Lunch

Meatballs In Tomato Gravy

Dinner

Stir Fried Zucchini

Day 27

Breakfast

Veggie Mash

Lunch

Shrimp & Veggies Curry

Dinner

Green Beans With Tomatoes

Day 28

Breakfast

Choco Banana Bites

Lunch

Shrimp With Zucchini

Dinner

Lamb Curry

Day 29

Breakfast

Mixed Veggie Salad

Lunch

Shrimp With Broccoli

Dinner

Grilled Salmon With Ginger Sauce

Day 30

Breakfast

Tofu Scramble

Lunch

Tortilla Chicken Soup

Dinner

Chicken Fajitas

www.ingramcontent.com/pod-product-compliance
Lightning Source LLC
LaVergne TN
LVHW082225230325
806688LV00005B/38